Preparticipa
Physical
Evaluation

MW01122557

THIRD EDITION

 American Academy of Family Physicians

 American Academy of Pediatrics

 American College of Sports Medicine

 American Medical Society for Sports Medicine

 American Orthopaedic Society for Sports Medicine

 American Osteopathic Academy of Sports Medicine

**Preparticipation Physical Evaluation
Working Group and Authors**

Gordon O. Matheson, MD, PhD (Facilitator)
Lori A. Boyajian-O'Neill, DO (AOASM)
Dennis Cardone, DO (AAFP)
William Dexter, MD (ACSM)
John DiFiori, MD (AMSSM)
K. Bert Fields, MD (AMSSM)
Deryk Jones, MD (AOSSM)
Robert Pallay, MD (AAFP)
Frederick Reed, Jr, MD (AAP)
William O. Roberts, MD (ACSM)
Eric Small, MD (AAP)
Randall Wroble, MD (AOSSM)
Phillip Zinni III, DO, ATC (AOASM)

The author societies wish to
acknowledge these individuals
for their exceptional contributions
to this project:

John J. Dougherty, DO
E. Randy Eichner, MD
Kristin Wingfield, MD

The McGraw-Hill Companies

**the
physician
and
sportsmedicine**

The Physician and Sportsmedicine
A division of the McGraw-Hill Companies
Minneapolis, New York City

McGraw-Hill Healthcare Information
The Physician and Sportsmedicine
4530 W 77th St
Minneapolis, MN 55435
To Order: 1-800-262-4729
Online Orders: http://books.mcgraw-hill.com/cgi-bin/pbg/0071446362

Executive Editor: James R. Wappes
Art Director: Jim Bauer
Illustrations: Terry Boles, Rebekah Dodson

The McGraw-Hill Companies

**the
physician
and
sportsmedicine**

Printed in the United States of America
Last digit is the print number: 9 8 7 6 5 4 3 2 1

ISBN 0-07-144636-2

Preparticipation Physical Evaluation

THIRD EDITION

National Endorsements of the Third Edition

- ◆ **Endorsed by the National Athletic Trainers' Association.**
- ◆ **Endorsed by the Sports Physical Therapy Section of the American Physical Therapy Association.**
- ◆ **Approved by the Special Olympics Medical Committee as meeting its standards for athletic participation.**

Acknowledgement: The Gatorade Sports Science Institute provided an unrestricted educational grant for funding a process meeting forum and a focus group in the production of this edition.

PREFACE

Although the preparticipation evaluation (PPE) has been frequently used in a variety of settings, there has not been a systematic approach to its development, implementation, or evaluation. Since publication of the first edition of the *Preparticipation Physical Evaluation* monograph in 1992, there have been multiple studies and much debate addressing the effectiveness of the PPE as a screening tool for athletic clearance. Criticism and concerns have been raised regarding the ability of the PPE to affect outcomes, such as predicting or preventing injury. In particular, the ability of the PPE to detect athletes at risk for potentially catastrophic events, such as sudden cardiac death from hypertrophic cardiomyopathy, has been questioned.

Despite these concerns, the author societies (American Academy of Family Physicians [AAFP], American Academy of Pediatrics [AAP], American College of Sports Medicine [ACSM], American Medical Society for Sports Medicine [AMSSM], American Orthopaedic Society for Sports Medicine [AOSSM], and American Osteopathic Academy of Sports Medicine [AOASM]) recognize the important role the PPE might play, primarily for screening athletes, but also in the overall provision of healthcare, particularly in the adolescent population.

This third edition reflects a rigorous attempt to identify and outline efficacious principles and practices in the PPE. The process included:

- Definition of the issues surrounding the PPE;
- An extensive review of the literature;
- Use of position, policy, and consensus statements from major organizations;
- Review of expert opinion;
- Focus-group feedback on the PPE process, questions, and forms;
- Extensive peer review by other experts from all the author societies (leading to multiple revisions); and
- Review by legal counsel.

This edition of *Preparticipation Physical Evaluation* has been reviewed even more extensively than the second edition, and we greatly appreciate the excellent recommendations of the many professionals from the 6 societies who have reviewed specific sections or the whole document. These individuals include experts in primary care and multiple specialties, both private practitioners and academicians.

The author societies hope that this guide will serve to enhance the health and safety of athletes and will make the PPE an enjoyable, informative, and useful experience for both practitioner and patient. In addition to facilitating care of the athlete, a standardized approach to the PPE will set the stage for data collection that may lead to future insights and changes based on outcomes.

TABLE OF CONTENTS

Acronyms Used in This Edition

Organizations

AAFP	American Academy of Family Physicians
AAP	American Academy of Pediatrics
ACSM	American College of Sports Medicine
AMSSM	American Medical Society for Sports Medicine
AOASM	American Osteopathic Academy of Sports Medicine
AOSSM	American Orthopaedic Society for Sports Medicine
AAN	American Academy of Neurology
AAO	American Academy of Ophthalmology
AHA	American Heart Association
AHIMA	American Health Information Management Association
AMA	American Medical Association
ANSI	American National Standards Institute
CDC	Centers for Disease Control and Prevention
FDA	Food and Drug Administration
HHS	Department of Health and Human Services
IOM	Institute of Medicine
NCAA	National Collegiate Athletic Association
NFHS	National Federation of State High School Associations
NFL	National Football League
NGB	National governing body
SAM	Society for Adolescent Medicine
USADA	United States Anti-Doping Agency
USPSTF	United States Preventive Services Task Force
WADA	World Anti-Doping Agency

Other Acronyms

PPE	Preparticipation evaluation
AAI	Atlantoaxial instability
BMI	Body mass index
CCN	Cervical cord neurapraxia
CI	Cognitively impaired
CT	Computed tomography
ECG	Electrocardiogram
e-HIM	Electronic health information management
EHR	Electronic health record
e-PPE	Electronic preparticipation evaluation
EIA	Exercise-induced asthma
EIB	Exercise-induced bronchoconstriction
FERPA	Family Education Rights and Privacy Act
FEV_1	Forced expiratory volume in 1 sec
FVC	Forced vital capacity
GAPS	Guidelines for Adolescent Preventive Services
HCM	Hypertrophic cardiomyopathy
HEENT	Head, eyes, ears, nose, and throat
HIPAA	Health Insurance Portability and Accountability Act
HBV	Hepatitis B virus
HCV	Hepatitis C virus
HIV	Human immunodeficiency virus
ICD	Implantable cardioverter defibrillator
MRI	Magnetic resonance imaging
MRSA	Methicillin-resistant *Staphylococcus aureus*
NAEPP	National Asthma Education and Prevention Program
PI	Physically impaired
RBC	Red blood cell
SIS	Second impact syndrome
YRBSS	Youth Risk Behavior Surveillance System

Chapter 1

INTRODUCTION

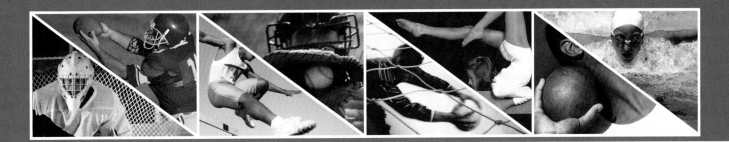

The overall goal in performing a preparticipation examination (PPE) is to promote the health and safety of the athlete in training and competition. The PPE is a tool to screen athletes for injuries, illness, or factors that might put them or others at risk. Ideally, it will also identify conditions that might interfere with optimal athletic performance and might require further investigation and/or treatment.

For a screening tool to be effective, it must meet several criteria. It must identify diseases or processes that will affect the athlete, be sensitive and accurate, and be practical and affordable. Currently, data on the ability of the PPE to meet these criteria are lacking. Despite this lack of efficacy data, the exams are widely performed. Almost all states require some level of PPE for scholastic athletes. The National Federation of State High School Associations (NFHS) considers the PPE a precondition to participation. At the collegiate level, the National Collegiate Athletic Association (NCAA) recommends, and most institutions require, a PPE at least on entrance to the program.[1,2] In addition, Special Olympics requires a PPE for its athletes (see "The Athlete With Special Needs," chapter 8, page 79).

Requirements regarding the PPE vary widely by state, locality, and institution and in content, length, and comprehensiveness. This variance is well illustrated by several studies that demonstrated that most PPE forms used in high school or college do not follow American Heart Association (AHA) guidelines regarding appropriate cardiac screening.[3-5] In a number of states, providers of varying levels of training and expertise are permitted to administer the PPE to athletes.[4] Equally wide variation exists in how physicians approach, conduct, and document these exams.

While acknowledging these concerns, the author societies agree that the PPE, when thoroughly and consistently performed and supervised by qualified and licensed physicians, can be an effective tool in identifying medical and orthopedic conditions that might affect an athlete's ability to participate safely in sports. The PPE also serves as an important component of adolescent healthcare.

The purpose of the PPE is to facilitate and encourage safe participation, not to exclude athletes from participation. While 1 systematic review[6] of the PPE (> 20,000 exams) found only 3 athletes that were excluded, most individual studies report that 0.3% to 1.3% of athletes are denied clearance to participate during the PPE, with 3.2% to 13.9% requiring further evaluation prior to participation.[4,7-12]

For many if not most adolescents, the PPE is their only contact with a medical provider in any given year.[3,8] While the PPE is not intended to substitute for athletes' regular health maintenance exams, it can provide an opportunity to facilitate general healthcare.

This monograph is intended to provide a "state-of-the-art," practical, and effective screening tool for physicians who perform PPEs for athletes in middle school, high school, and college. It is designed for use as a stand-alone screening exam that can be easily incorporated into routine preventive examinations. The process and forms are designed to apply in most settings (office, school, urban, rural) and are easily adaptable to suit individual or institutional needs.

This third edition includes descriptions of goals, objectives, timing, setting, and structure of the exam; details the history and physical examination; lists return-to-play-guidelines; and addresses medicolegal concerns. The text of the monograph reviews the rationale for the primary and secondary history questions as well as the examination maneuvers. Numerous references are provided, including Web sites, to support the discussion, provide useful resources, and offer a basis for further inquiry. New sections include particulars for athletes with special needs, administrative concerns, and future directions. Succinct, comprehensive, easily used forms (pages 93 through 95) are supplied for athletes, parents, and clinicians.

REFERENCES

1. Montalto NJ: Implementing the guidelines for adolescent preventive services. Am Fam Physician 1998;57(9):2181-2190
2. MacAuley D: Does preseason screening for cardiac disease really work? the British perspective. Med Sci Sports Exerc 1998;30(10 suppl):S345-S350
3. Krowchuk DP, Krowchuk HV, Hunter M, et al: Parents' knowledge of the purposes and content of preparticipation physical examinations. Arch Pediatr Adolesc Med 1995;149(6):653-657
4. Fuller CM: Cost effectiveness analysis of screening of high school athletes for risk of sudden cardiac death. Med Sci Sports Exerc 2000;32(5) 887-890
5. Glover DW, Maron BJ: Profile of preparticipation cardio-vascular screening for high school athletes. JAMA 1998;279(22):1817-1819
6. Stickler GB: Are yearly physical examinations in adolescents necessary? J Am Board Fam Pract 2000;13(3):172-177
7. Klein JD, Slap GB, Elster AB, et al: Access to health care for adolescents: position paper of the Society for Adolescent Medicine. J Adolesc Health 1992;13(2):162-170
8. Carek PJ, Futrell M: Athletes' view of the preparticipation physical examination. Arch Fam Med 1999;8(4):307-312
9. Rosen DS, Elster A, Hedberg V, et al: Clinical preventive services for adolescents: position paper of the Society for Adolescent Medicine. J Adolesc Health 1997;21(3):203-214
10. Fuller CM, McNulty CM, Spring DA, et al: Prospective screening of 5,615 high school athletes for risk of sudden cardiac death. Med Sci Sports Exerc 1997;29(9):1131-1138
11. Lyznicki JM, Nielsen NH: Cardiovascular screening of student athletes. Am Fam Physician 2000;62(4):765-774
12. Koester MC, Amundson CL: Preparticipation screening of high school athletes: are recommendations enough? Phys Sportsmed 2003;31(8):35-38

Chapter 2
GOALS AND OBJECTIVES

T he overall goal of the PPE is achieved by adhering to the primary objectives (table 1). The secondary objectives take advantage of the opportunity provided by the athlete's contact with the physician (and healthcare system) during the PPE (see table 1). Ultimately, the PPE provides the medical background on which decisions will be made by the team physician and medical staff. It is well documented that 75% or more of medical and orthopedic conditions are detected by the history alone.[1-3] This monograph focuses on the history as the most relevant aspect of the PPE. Where possible, the forms include validated questions (eg, from the Youth Risk Behavioral Survey). Recommendations from consensus documents by other organizations, such as the AHA and the United States Preventive Services Task Force (USPSTF), have also been used.

■ PRIMARY OBJECTIVES

1. Detect potentially life-threatening or disabling medical or musculoskeletal conditions. Both absolute and relative contraindications are considered. For example, myocarditis is an absolute contraindication for any sport because of the risk of sudden death with exertion. Ventricular septal defect, however, is a relative contraindication, because the athlete may be able to participate, depending on the severity of the defect. There is no solid evidence that a screening PPE will reliably identify important but clinically silent conditions (such as hypertrophic cardiomyopathy), yet the consensus panel feels that a comprehensive approach to the PPE uniformly applied seems to offer the best opportu-

Table 1	**Objectives of the PPE**

Primary Objectives
1. Screen for conditions that may be life-threatening or disabling
2. Screen for conditions that may predispose to injury or illness
3. Meet administrative requirements

Secondary Objectives
1. Determine general health
2. Serve as an entry point to the healthcare system for adolescents
3. Provide opportunity to initiate discussion on health-related topics

nity to meet this objective.

2. Screen for medical or musculoskeletal conditions that may predispose an athlete to injury or illness during training or competition. In 1 survey[2] of 716 athletes, about 66% believed that the PPE was not absolutely necessary to participate safely in sports. However, more than 90% believed that the PPE could help prevent injury. Though evidence is lacking regarding the PPE's ability to conclusively meet this objective, there is general agreement that identification of conditions that may predispose an athlete to injury or illness is worthwhile. Such conditions include acute, recurrent, chronic, or untreated injuries or illnesses, inadequately rehabilitated injuries, and congenital or developmental problems.

Early recognition of any of these problems minimizes time lost from play by allowing initiation of evaluation and treatment and completion of rehabilitation. For example, an obese athlete is at an increased risk for heat illness and may benefit from counseling on weight control, acclimatization, and hydration before the season starts. Similarly, an athlete with recurrent ankle sprains who has returned to sports prior to completing ankle rehabilitation will likely benefit from instruction and follow-up regarding appropriate rehabilitation. Identification of those with exercise-induced asthma allows the physician to initiate treatment or refer the athlete for appropriate care.

3. Address administrative requirements. States, school districts, institutions, and organizations have their own regulations and requirements concerning eligibility for participation for student-athletes. Federal mandates exist (eg, the Americans With Disabilities Act, Health Insurance Portability and Accountability Act [HIPAA], and Family Education Rights and Privacy Act [FERPA]; see "Administrative and Legal Concerns," chapter 4, page 11) that address a range of athlete rights from confidentiality to participation. The physician must be aware of, and take into account, these concerns in providing PPE services to athletes.

■ SECONDARY OBJECTIVES

1. Determine general health. Studies have shown that adolescents are less likely than any other age-group to see a healthcare provider. In fact, the only contact most will have with the healthcare system is via a required PPE.[4] This finding may be especially true of athletes from low-income families who cannot afford routine medical care. One review of the effectiveness of the PPE in identifying abnormalities suggests that yearly examinations of adolescents are not useful or cost effective.[5] However, the Society for Adolescent Medicine (SAM) estimates that 5% to 10% of adolescents will have a chronic condition that requires ongoing care, and up to half of adolescents will have less severe medical problems.[6] Furthermore, there are other reasons to consider periodic health exams including screening, counseling, and establishing a "medical home" or relationship. The Guidelines for Adolescent Preventive Services (GAPS) developed by the American Medical Association (AMA) and the Centers for Disease Control and Prevention (CDC) recommends that all adolescents have an annual routine health exam. A similar recommendation is made by the SAM, AAP, AAFP, and USPSTF.[7,8]

2. Serve as entry point into the healthcare system for adolescents. The SAM recommends that healthcare for adolescents be readily available, visible, confidential, affordable, and flexible.[9] A thorough PPE can and ideally should be integrated into a regular examination with the athlete's personal physician. It is not intended to replace these visits. However, since the PPE is the only periodic health examination for many athletes, it seems prudent to acknowledge the reality of how and when adolescents receive healthcare.

One interesting study[3] notes that up to one third of parents identify the PPE as their student-athlete's only contact with the healthcare system—even when up to 90% had an identified primary care provider and their insurance covered yearly health maintenance exams. While 95% of parents agreed with the primary goals of the PPE (to detect conditions that might affect participation) and 68% believed it should be minimal, one-third thought the PPE should address other health issues and might be a reasonable alternative to routine comprehensive exams.

Given the above, and viewing the PPE as a point of entry to the healthcare system, follow-up becomes a critical component of the PPE process. Special attention must be paid to having a careful system to generate necessary referrals; particularly for PPEs not done one-on-one in the private physician's office.

3. Provide opportunity for discussion on health and lifestyle issues. The opportunity to use the PPE as a way to engage adolescents in a discussion on health issues should not be overlooked. There is little evidence that supports brief counseling interventions with adolescent lifestyle issues (eg, tobacco and alcohol consumption), but the AAP and SAM recommend such counseling for preventive visits. The PPE provides an opportunity to begin this dialogue.

Seventy percent of adolescents express a desire for more healthcare information from their physician. Despite this statistic, most adolescents also relate that they are not comfortable with questions related to risk behaviors, substance use, sexuality, or weight and diet in the context of a station-based exam.[6] Depending on available time, the PPE, particularly when performed as an office-based or perhaps a modified one-on-one coordinated medical team examination (see page 7), may provide an opportunity for counseling the athlete and answering health-related questions if comfort and reasonable confidentiality are ensured.

Issues that arise may include an explanation of abnormal findings or topics such as proper training techniques, weight-control behaviors, and nutrition. Tobacco use, drinking and driving, drug use, seat belt use, prevention of sexually transmitted diseases, and birth control may also be discussed. This objective may be hard to meet but should be attempted when practical. The information obtained during the PPE can provide the physician a means to at least initiate discussion with the athlete, or make appropriate referral for health-related and lifestyle issues.

REFERENCES

1. Koester MC, Amundson CL: Preparticipation screening of high school athletes: are recommendations enough? Phys Sportsmed 2003;31(8):35-38
2. Carek PJ, Futrell M: Athletes' view of the preparticipation physical examination. Arch Fam Med 1999;8(4):307-312
3. Krowchuk DP, Krowchuk HV, Hunter M, et al: Parents' knowledge of the purposes and content of preparticipation physical examinations. Arch Pediatr Adolesc Med 1995;149(6):653-657
4. Metzl, JD: The adolescent preparticipation physical examination: is it helpful? Clin Sports Med 2000;19(4):577-590
5. Montalto NJ: Implementing the guidelines for adolescent preventive services. Am Fam Physician 1998;57(9):2181-2190
6. Klein JD, Slap GB, Elster AB, et al: Access to health care for adolescents: position paper of the Society for Adolescent Medicine. J Adolesc Health 1992;13(2):162-170
7. Medical evaluations, immunizations and records, in: NCAA Sports Medicine Handbook, ed 16. Indianapolis, National Collegiate Athletic Association, 2003, p 8
8. United States Preventive Services Task Force: The Guide to Medical Prevention Services, ed 2. Alexandria, VA, International Medical Publishing Inc, 1996
9. Rosen DS, Elster A, Hedberg V, et al: Clinical preventive services for adolescents: position paper of the Society for Adolescent Medicine. J Adolesc Health 1997;21(3):203-214

Chapter 3

TIMING, SETTING, AND STRUCTURE

◣ QUALIFICATIONS OF THE EXAMINERS

Physicians who have earned an MD or DO have training and an unrestricted medical license that allows them to deal with the broad range of problems that may be encountered during the PPE. For this reason, the PPE working group concurs that the ultimate responsibility for the PPE should be assigned to an MD or DO physician.[1-3] Physicians desiring to perform PPEs must fulfill the goals and objectives outlined in the previous section and should use consultation to address problems beyond their expertise.[1]

State regulations determine which practitioners are licensed to perform PPEs for public middle and high schools. Many states allow healthcare professionals other than physicians to perform the evaluation. Regardless of their training, practitioners performing PPEs should competently screen athletes for the type of problems that would affect participation or place the athlete at undue risk. At the collegiate, professional, national, and international competition levels, the respective athletic governing bodies determine who may perform the PPE.

When PPEs are done in a group setting, the team physician should coordinate the process and supervise a team of healthcare professionals to ensure that all appropriate components of the assessment take place[4] (table 2).

◣ TIMING OF THE EVALUATION

To allow time to treat or rehabilitate any identified problem, the PPE should ideally be performed at least 6 weeks prior to preseason practice. The PPE working group feels that student-athletes should schedule this with their personal physician, who has access to medical records and can adjust treatment of chronic medical conditions. Good options include scheduling PPEs in midsummer or even at the end of the previous school year. This approach allows the student-athlete to deal with issues when they will have less impact on school attendance and sports practice. Student-athletes need clear information about how to handle PPE forms so that although the school receives clearance forms, the medical record remains confidential and can be accessed only by designated medical providers and in accordance with HIPAA (see "Administrative and Legal Concerns," chapter 4, page 11).

Athletes examined at the end of the school year for a sport occurring the next fall should be questioned by the team physician and/or athletic trainers prior to fall practice to allow evaluation of any injuries or illnesses that occurred during the summer. College sports medicine programs coordinate the PPE screening process to have these exams completed before the student-athletes begin practice in their respective sports.

Table 2	Elements of a Coordinated Medical Evaluation

Stage	Purpose
Waiting area	Sign-in, registration, and review, including careful instruction about filling out required forms
Vitals station	Height, weight,* blood pressure, vision
Office examination	History review, physical examination performed by 1 physician for a given student-athlete
Specialty offices	Orthopedic assessment, cardiology evaluation, etc
Optional stages	Educational and rehabilitation areas

*Body mass index can be calculated from height and weight (see www.cdc.gov/growthcharts).

◤ FREQUENCY OF THE EVALUATION

Colleges generally determine the policies that their athletic departments mandate for PPEs. Since college students typically attend school away from their parents and their personal physicians, more comprehensive health examinations at entry into a collegiate athletic program are the norm. Once a comprehensive evaluation has occurred, student-athletes undergo briefer yearly examinations that focus on any injuries and illnesses that occurred after the comprehensive examination. The team physician at the collegiate level needs to become familiar with the health history of the student-athletes and typically will perform many of the examinations as well as reviewing information from all those done. This PPE working group feels this frequency is appropriate for the college age-group.[1]

At the secondary school level, review of PPEs from the various states reveals that 2 main options are currently used. Most states require a yearly examination with a mandated form. Other states require completion of a more comprehensive PPE at the entrance to middle or high school, followed by completion of an annual form that updates injuries or illnesses over the past year.

Significant issues have delayed implementation of a nationwide format for PPEs or even a standard recommendation regarding frequency. Factors that have influenced these decisions include: (1) requirements of specific schools or states; (2) the degree of risk of a particular sport; (3) cost, especially out-of-pocket expenses for students, since these will be barriers to participation; and (4) availability of qualified personnel.

No outcome-based research indicates that more frequent PPEs lessen the risk of injury or death in student-athletes, so an optimal frequency for the examination has not been established.[4-12] The consensus of the PPE working group is:

◆ A comprehensive PPE should be performed every 2 years in younger student-athletes and every 2 to 3 years in older athletes.

◆ A comprehensive PPE should occur at entry into middle school and high school or upon transfer to a new school.

◆ Annual updates should include a comprehensive history, height, weight, blood pressure, and a problem-focused examination of any concerns detected in the history.

The basis for this recommendation is that younger student-athletes pass through stages of adolescent development that have both physiologic and psychological changes that merit monitoring. Careful cardiac auscultation on an every-other-year basis may help screen for unknown cardiac conditions. The annual history review also allows an opportunity to detect those athletes who have new concerns or injuries since the time of their comprehensive exam.

One key argument for performing a complete PPE annually is that many athletes and parents plan to use the PPE as their only visit for healthcare.[13] However, when student-athletes have no primary physician, the PPE is unlikely to be an adequate opportunity to address all of their healthcare. With this in mind, the examining physician should encourage the student-athlete to establish care with a primary care physician. Conversely, when the student-athlete's personal physician performs annual examinations, required elements of the PPE can be incorporated along with continuity of care and health education, and a separate visit for a PPE would not be needed. Incorporating the PPE into the routine healthcare screening schedule after age 6 can help promote physical activity and sports safety in children and adolescents.

◤ METHODS AND SETTING OF EVALUATIONS

The most common methods for performing PPEs are individual examinations or assessments by a coordinated medical team. The settings for the PPE are in the physician's office or a similar private setting. The PPE working group considers "gymnasium examinations" as inappropriate to accomplish the goals and objectives of the PPE process. Since most student-athletes are adolescents, parents should not be in the room for the full PPE so that the physician can inquire about adolescent risk behaviors. When a group of medical personnel work together to complete the PPE, the key portion of the process should still be a one-on-one examination with a physician.

The primary care physician's office for the PPE allows better continuity of care. The student-athlete's personal physician, who has an established relationship, is likely to know the patient's history and have a complete set of medical records, including family history, immunizations, and laboratory studies. This reduces the possibility that an abnormality will be missed and predispose an athlete to unnecessary risk. The personal physician is also less likely to overlook something that was inadvertently or consciously omitted during completion of the preparticipation history form.

In addition, for student-athletes with known medical problems, the personal physician should have a better sense of the stability of the condition and can make changes in treatment that should allow safer participation. If needed, the personal physician can also coordinate with families to see that appropriate consultations are arranged. The PPE working group believes that this is the ideal place to have the PPE completed.

The office setting typically offers privacy and a chance to discuss confidential issues. Familiarity also provides an opportunity to counsel the athlete on sensitive issues such as alcohol and drug use, birth control, and prevention of sexually transmitted diseases. Young athletes are far more willing to discuss these issues with someone they trust.

For personal physicians to play a greater role in the PPE process, both student-athletes and parents must assume greater responsibility for having the PPE completed. This includes taking the initiative to schedule an appointment to the physician's office well before the start of the sport season. Athletes who wait until the week before their season starts aren't likely to be cleared in time.

Coordinated medical team examinations have a useful role, particularly for student-athletes who do not have a personal physician or may have consulted different specialists for prior medical problems. Often these exams are done as a community service and can reduce cost for student-athletes who have limited financial resources. In addition, this setting may be preferred when the student-athlete's personal physician does not feel comfortable determining clearance or evaluating specific conditions that may predispose the athlete to further injury or illness. Coordinated medical teams typically are organized by the team physician and often involve both primary care and orthopedic sports medicine specialists. Other medical specialists and professionals may allow on-site evaluation of a wide range of problems.

In the coordinated medical team approach in which multiple physicians are involved (table 3), the PPE working group recommends that 1 physician review the history and perform the exam for a student-athlete. However, on review of the history form, individ-

Table 3	Tips to Improve the Coordinated Medical Team Approach to PPEs

Provide athletes in advance with information about the detailed nature of the examination and the appropriate attire to wear to lessen privacy concerns and increase efficiency*

Ensure separate areas for examining male and female athletes

Have a private individual counseling room for discussion of sensitive issues to maintain confidentiality and facilitate better communication

Enhance familiarity and continuity of care by enlisting the assistance of as many primary physicians as possible for the athletes being examined

Establish a clear protocol for referral to primary physicians, specialists, rehabilitation, or other medical evaluations for every student-athlete who is not cleared for participation because of illness or injury. Athletes from low-income families, in particular, may need help in arranging and completing follow-up evaluations. If there is a team physician, he or she should keep—and follow up on—a list of athletes who are disqualified or who require further evaluation before final clearance (see "Determining Clearance," chapter 7, page 61). If the athlete is not cleared for the desired sport, the evaluating physician should counsel the athlete concerning alternate permissible activities.

*Filling out the history, physical examination, and clearance forms (pages 93-95) carefully can improve the entire process. Therefore, at the start of a coordinated medical team evaluation, explaining to the student-athletes how to correctly complete the forms will result in a more useful completed form. Appropriate privacy, storage, and handling of forms can give the athlete greater confidence in the confidentiality of the process.

uals with known medical issues could be directed to the primary care physicians, and those with known orthopedic issues could be primarily screened by the orthopedists. By working as a medical team, physicians can also rely on colleagues to help with difficult assessments rather than having to refer as often. This approach becomes essential in some more rural settings where limited availability of primary care physicians may delay the process. Colleges typically use a coordinated medical team and may institute special evaluations uniquely useful for a given sport.

Effective coordination of PPEs requires assembling the right mix of personnel. There must be adequate numbers of physicians to comprehensively review each PPE. Primary care and orthopedic physicians can complement each other's skills in this setting, and subspecialty physicians such as cardiologists can play a useful role within their particular area of expertise. Physical therapists, athletic trainers, nutritionists, and exercise physiologists can be incorporated to help with patient education and teaching of rehabilitation exercises. The team physician typically can't screen all individuals but, by coordinating the process, can learn the overall health status of many student-athletes and be brought into the evaluation of all those with serious problems.

The team physician must choose a location that will allow adequate space for large number of participants while at the same time ensuring privacy and preventing the noise and confusion that often arise in a gymnasium. A number of physicians use their medical offices after hours to conduct these exams so that individual examiners and athletes have privacy. The rooms can still be arranged to allow specific consultations to take place.

When a student-athlete merits disqualification, good communication between the evaluating physician, the student-athlete, and the athlete's parent(s) or guardian(s) is essential. In the medical team setting, the team physician can take part in this discussion, often leading it.

◤ INTERIM ANNUAL EVALUATIONS

An annual evaluation takes place between comprehensive examinations. To complete this evaluation, all student-athletes should answer a comprehensive history questionnaire; have their height, weight, and blood pressure recorded; and undergo any focused examination indicated by the history. The purpose of the interim evaluation is to assess problems that have occurred since the athlete's full PPE. This also serves as a time to reinforce previously discussed lifestyle issues and restate critical questions regarding syncope and concussion that athletes have been known to answer in a way to avoid disqualification.

The physician reviews the history form and determines what parts of the physical examination should be performed. While this may be a very brief visit, if the physician identifies potentially serious symptoms such as a student-athlete with syncope during exercise, a complete cardiovascular assessment would be required before clearance is granted.

◤ ROUTINE SCREENING TESTS

Routine laboratory, cardiac, and pulmonary screening tests for PPEs remain controversial. However, since evidenced-based studies to indicate their utility are lacking, the PPE working group concurs that no routine screening tests are required for the PPE of asymptomatic athletes.

This judgment hinges on the difference between screening and diagnostic tests. The value of a screening test or procedure depends on two variables: (1) the predictive value of the proposed screen, which is in turn affected by the prevalence of the condition in the population being screened, and (2) the ability to reduce morbidity and mortality by identifying the condition with the screening method. The screening test must also be acceptable in terms of cost and potential side effects. The value of a diagnostic test, on the other hand, is in its ability to pinpoint a condition for which suspicion already exists by history or physical examination.

When evaluating screening tests with the aforementioned criteria, studies have not supported the use of such tests as urinalysis, complete blood count, chemistry profile, lipid profile, ferritin level, or sickle cell trait in the PPE.[14-18] Similarly, cardiopulmonary testing with electrocardiogram (ECG), echocardiogram, exercise stress testing, or spirometry lacks research to demonstrate that it clearly meets these criteria either.[19-25]

Cardiac screening remains controversial: Authors have advocated the use of screening ECGs and screening echocardiograms (usually limited to septum and free posterior left ventricular wall) to improve our ability to identify athletes at risk of sudden cardiac death.[26,27] However, at best we have indirect evidence that noninvasive cardiovascular screening could potentially identify conditions such as hypertrophic cardiomyopathy (HCM).[28,29] On the other hand, no outcome-based studies have identified that these tests can consistently identify the high-risk athlete or reduce the incidence of sudden cardiac death.

In addition, cardiac tests generate false-positive results that require complete evaluation and expensive testing to rule out cardiovascular disease. ECG and echocardiographic studies yield mixed results, with better identification of high-risk individuals when the tests are used for directed cardiovascular evaluation rather than general screening.[20-23,29-31]

The PPE working group acknowledges the importance of better cardiovascular screening. It also recognizes, however, that a test that detects the 1:100,000 to 1:300,000 athletes at risk for sudden cardiac death[32,33] would have to demonstrate high sensitivity and specificity to merit the cost of implementation into a nationwide PPE process.

Exercise-induced asthma (EIA) is such a common problem that a good screen during the PPE would have great utility. EIA prevalence varies by sport and environmental conditions. For example, recent screens of elite runners revealed 10% of the men and 26% of the women had EIA.[34] Screens for winter sports have demonstrated positive tests for approximately 50% of figure skaters[35-38] and 79% of cross-country skiers.[39] The prevalence of EIA in high school, collegiate, and Olympic athletes is estimated as high as 20%, with a significant number of these athletes undiagnosed.

However, a satisfactory screen for EIA has yet to be demonstrated. Although a history of cough with exercise or allergic rhinitis—or a family history of asthma—identifies individuals at higher risk, additional studies have shown that the history, physical examination, and resting spirometry are not reliable enough to identify the athlete who has EIA.[24,25,40,41] Exercise challenge tests or eucapnic hyperventilation tests, both of which are more sensitive than the history and physical examination alone, may be necessary to identify the disorder.[24,25,41,42] However, unless large studies indicate that these tests can efficiently and inexpensively be incorporated into the PPE, they are not likely to be recommended.

Findings from the medical history or physical exam may indicate a need to arrange specific diagnostic tests. For example, a complete hematologic profile may be recommended to check for anemia or nutritional deficiency in an athlete who has fatigue, pallor, performance decline, heavy menstrual bleeding, low calorie intake, or a diet lacking red meat. A lipid profile to test for familial dyslipidemia is recommended in a student-athlete who has a family history of premature atherosclerotic heart disease or dyslipidemia. Urinalysis may be indicated in an athlete with dysuria, hematuria, or a family history of certain types of kidney disease. The examining physician decides clearance for sports participation while awaiting completion of diagnostic testing, but specific recommendations for testing for various conditions are not standardized as a part of the screening examination.

Urine drug screening and human immunodeficiency virus (HIV) screening deserve mention. Routine urine drug testing at the elite amateur and professional levels is now fairly common and is becoming more widely used in Division 1 college athletics. Mandatory HIV testing is discouraged because of the low risk of transmission, although certain boxing organizations require it.[43,44]

Physicians performing PPEs should be familiar with the screening test guidelines established by the athletic governing body under which the athlete competes. Nevertheless, physicians must exercise caution and also consider the medical, legal, and confidentiality issues that drug screening and HIV testing entail. Furthermore, if drug screening or HIV testing is implemented, a formal plan for secure sample collection and an institutional policy for dealing with positive tests must be established.

While mandatory testing of athletes for HIV or hepatitis is not recommended,[45,46] voluntary testing should be encouraged for athletes who have exposure to blood products, symptoms suggestive of disease, or significant risk factors detected during the PPE. Risk factors include: (1) multiple sex partners; (2) sexual contact with infected individuals; (3) blood transfusions before 1985; (4) sexually transmitted diseases, including hepatitis B virus; (5) a history of intravenous drug abuse or injections of ergogenic drugs, or use of such drugs by sexual partners; (6) male homosexuality; and, (7) in girls, bisexual partners.[46]

REFERENCES

1. Team physician consensus statement. Med Sci Sports Exerc 2000;32(4):877-878
2. Team physician consensus statement. Am J Sports Med 2000;28(3):440-441
3. Sideline preparedness for the team physician: a consensus statement. Med Sci Sports Exerc 2001;33(5):846-849
4. American Academy of Family Physicians, American Academy of Pediatrics, American Medical Society for Sports Medicine, American Orthopaedic Society for Sports Medicine, American Osteopathic Academy of Sports Medicine: Preparticipation Physical Evaluation, ed 2. Minneapolis, New York City, McGraw-Hill Inc, 1997
5. Wingfield K, Matheson GO, Meeuwisse WH: Preparticipation evaluation: an evidence-based review. Clin J Sport Med 2004;14(3):109-122
6. Brukner P, White S, Shawdon A, et al: Screening of athletes: Australian experience. Clin J Sport Med 2004;14(3):169-177
7. Rich BSE: Preparticipation physical examinations, ACSM Current Comment, 1999. Available at http://www.acsm.org/health+fitness/comments.htm. Accessed July 15, 2004
8. ICSI Health Care Guidelines: Preventing counseling and education. Available at http://www.icsi.org/knowledge/detail.asp?catID=29&itemID=188. Accessed July 15, 2004
9. Metzl JD: Preparticipation examinations of the adolescent athlete, part 1. Pediatr Rev 2001;22(6):199-204
10. Stickler GB: Are yearly physical examinations in adolescents necessary? J Am Board Fam Pract 2000;13(3):172-177
11. O'Connor FG, Kugler JP, Oriscello RG: Sudden death in young athletes: screening for the needle in a haystack. Am Fam Physician 1998;57(11):2763-2770
12. Montalto NJ: Implementing the guidelines for adolescent preventive services. Am Fam Physician 1998;57(9):2181-2190
13. Krowchuk DP, Krowchuk HV, Hunter DM, et al: Parents' knowledge of the purpose and content of preparticipation physical examinations. Arch Pediatr Adolesc Med 1995;149(6):653-657
14. Lombardo JA, Robinson JB, Smith DM, et al: Preparticipation Physical Evaluation, ed 1. Kansas City, MO, American Academy of Family Physicians, American Academy of Pediatrics, American Medical Society for Sports Medicine, American Orthopaedic Society for Sports Medicine, American Osteopathic Academy of Sports Medicine, 1992
15. Dodge WF, West EF, Smith EH, et al: Proteinuria and hematuria in school children: epidemiology and early natural history. J Pediatr 1976;88(2):327-347
16. Peggs JF, Reinhardt RW, O'Brien JM: Proteinuria in adolescent sports physical examinations. J Fam Pract 1986;22(1):80-81
17. Taylor WC III, Lombardo JA: Preparticipation screening of college athletes: value of the complete blood cell count. Phys Sportsmed 1990;18(6):106-118
18. Vehaskari VM, Rapola J: Isolated proteinuria: analysis of a school-age population. J Pediact 1982;101(5):661-668
19. Ades PA: Preventing sudden death: cardiovascular screening of young athletes. Phys Sportsmed 1992;20(9):75-89
20. Epstein SE, Maron BJ: Sudden death and the competitive athlete: perspectives on preparticipation screening studies. J Am Coll Cardiol 1986;7(1):220-230
21. Feinstein RA, Colvin E, Oh MK: Echocardiographic screening as part of a preparticipation examination. Clin J Sport Med 1993;3(3):149-152
22. Lewis JF, Maron BJ, Diggs JA, et al: Preparticipation echocardiographic screening for cardiovascular disease in a large, predominantly black population of collegiate athletes. Am J Cardiol 1989;64(16):1029-1033
23. Maron BJ, Bodison SA, Wesley YE, et al: Results of screening a large group of intercollegiate competitive athletes for cardio-vascular disease. J Am Coll Cardiol 1987;10(6):1214-1221
24. Rupp NT, Brudno DS, Guill MF: The value of screening for risk of exercise-induced asthma in high school athletes. Ann Allergy 1993;70(4):339-342
25. Rupp NT, Guill MF, Brudno DS: Unrecognized exercise-induced bronchospasm in adolescent athletes. Am J Dis Child 1992;146(8):941-944
26. Fuller CM: Cost effectiveness analysis of screening of high school athletes for risk of sudden cardiac death. Med Sci Sports Exerc 2000;32(5):887-890
27. Fuller CM, McNutty CM, Spring DA, et al: Prospective screening of 5,615 high school athletes for risk of sudden cardiac death. Med Sci Sports Exerc 1997;29(9):1131-1138
28. Weidenbener EJ, Krauss MD, Waller BF, et al: Incorporation of screening echocardiography in the preparticipation exam. Clin J Sport Med 1995;5(2):86-89
29. Corrado D, Basso C, Schiavon M, et al: Screening for hyper-trophic cardiomyopathy in young athletes. N Engl J Med 1998;339(6):364-369
30. Maron BJ: Medical progress: Sudden death in young athletes. N Engl J Med 2003;349(11):1064-1075
31. Glover DW, Maron BJ: Profile of preparticipation cardiovascular screening for high school athletes. JAMA 1998;279 (22):1817-1819
32. Maron BJ, Shirani J, Poliac LC, et al: Sudden death in young competitive athletes: clinical, demographic, and pathological profiles. JAMA 1996;276(3):199-204
33. Van Camp SP, Bloor CM, Mueller FO, et al: Nontraumatic sports death in high school and college athletes. Med Sci Sports Exerc 1995;27(5):641-647
34. Schoene RB, Giboney K, Schimmel C, et al: Spirometry and airway reactivity in elite track and field athletes. Clin J Sport Med 1997;7(4):257-261
35. Mannix ET, Manfredi F, Farber MO: A comparison of two challenge tests for identifying exercise-induced broncho-spasm in figure skaters. Chest 1999;115(3):649-653
36. Provost-Craig MA, Arbour KS, Sestili DC, et al: The incidence of exercise-induced bronchospasm in competitive figure skaters. J Asthma 1996;33(1):67-71
37. Mannix ET, Farber MO, Palange P, et al: Exercise-induced asthma in figure skaters. Chest 1996;109(2):312-315
38. Wilber RL, Rundell KW, Szmedra L, et al: Incidence of exercise-induced bronchospasm in Olympic winter sport athletes. Med Sci Sports Exerc 2000;32(4);732-737
39. Larsson K, Ohlsen P, Larsson L, et al: High prevalence of asthma in cross country skiers. BMJ 1993:307(6915):1326-1329
40. Shield S, Wang-Dohlman A: Incidence of exercise-induced bronchospasm in high school football players, abstracted. J Allerg Clin Immunol 1991;87(1 pt 2 suppl):S166
41. Feinstein RA, LaRussa J, Wang-Dohlman A, et al: Screening adolescent athletes for exercised-induced asthma. Clin J Sport Med 1996;6(2):119-123
42. Holzer K, Brukner P: Screening of athletes for exercise-induced bronchospasm. Clin J Sport Med 2004;14(3):134-138
43. Mast EE, Goodman RA, Bond WW, et al: Transmission of blood-borne pathogens during sports: risk and prevention. Ann Intern Med 1995;122(4):283-285
44. Drotman DP: Professional boxing, bleeding, and HIV testing. JAMA 1996;276(3):193
45. Mitten MJ: HIV-positive athletes: when medicine meets the law. Phys Sportsmed 1994;22(10):63-68
46. American Medical Society for Sports Medicine, American Academy of Sports Medicine: Human immunodeficiency virus and other blood-borne pathogens in sports. Clin J Sport Med 1995;5(3):199-204

Chapter 4

ADMINISTRATIVE AND LEGAL CONCERNS

Physicians face several administrative and legal issues surrounding the PPE process, such as an athlete seeking to participate despite medical restrictions, real or perceived breaches of professional conduct during the exam, and the ramifications of Good Samaritan laws. Also, confidentiality and regulations regarding disclosure of medical information are as important with the PPE as with any medical interaction. And physicians may be asked to determine eligibility for the physically or cognitively impaired.

These issues are addressed in this section, but this chapter is not a legal opinion. It is intended as an overview of the issues pertaining to the PPE and athlete clearance for participation.

◣ RIGHT TO PARTICIPATE

Physicians delivering medical advice in the office setting based on data from a preparticipation exam have the same liability risks associated with any office exam and must always act in the best interest of the athlete. The clearance form has a "not cleared for certain sports or for all sports" check-off that will allow the physician to transmit the recommendation about a permanent disorder to the school without breaking the confidentiality rules that govern medical interactions.

Occasionally, the adage "first, do no harm" conflicts with the athlete's desire to compete when PPE findings lead to a recommendation for "no participation" in the athlete's sport. Although conditions that preclude participation are rare and many are well described, athletes will sometimes challenge activity restrictions, and the physician is confronted with an ethical dilemma that pits "informed choice" against "do no harm." Athletes may seek another medical opinion or pursue legal intervention to allow participation, even when accepted preparticipation recommendations like those of the AHA state that the risk is too great for safe play. The decision to restrict participation is not always clear-cut, and it is important to remember that these decisions are life-altering for affected athletes.

Ideally, the physician who advises restricted participation should seek the opinion of consulting physicians to develop a participation recommendation that reflects the relative risk for the athlete's safety during practice and competition. Following the consultations, it is imperative that the physician fully inform the athlete (and parents) of any risks associated with participation based on the disqualifying condition. This will allow the athlete and parents to make an informed decision regarding participation. Such discussions should be clearly documented in the athlete's medical record.

Federal enactments, such as the Rehabilitation Act of 1973 and the Americans With Disabilities Act of 1990, may allow an athlete with certain conditions the legal right to participate against medical advice.[1] Even when the recommendations published by major medical organizations strongly suggest restriction from activities due to the risk of sudden cardiac death, the courts have at times ruled against the restrictions placed on activity by a team physician as a result of the PPE findings.[2] Court decisions aside, sports organizations should stand behind the medical opinion if our system of preparticipation clearance for sports activity is to remain relevant.

Exculpatory waivers. If an athlete wishes to participate despite contrary medical recommendations, the athlete and his or her parent(s) or guardian(s) may suggest an "exculpatory waiver" or "risk release" to clearly indicate that they are fully informed of the inherent risk of participation against medical advice and that they assume this risk. If the athlete is under the age of majority, his or her parent(s) or guardian(s) must sign the waiver, and the physician must be aware of the age of majority in his or her state.

An exculpatory waiver or risk release is a written contract between the athlete and his or her parent(s) or guardian(s), the physician, and the school or activity sponsor. In it, the athlete promises not to sue the physician or activity sponsor and releases the physician and activity sponsor from liability.[3] However, the validity of these waivers may vary from state to state, and some legal experts question whether exculpatory waivers will adequately protect physicians from lawsuits.[4] Legal counsel for the sport sponsor and the physician is recommended on a case-by-case basis.

A physician may choose to allow an athlete to participate if the athlete and parents are willing to assume risk for a potentially catastrophic condition. To protect themselves, some legal experts recommend that the physician have the parents and athlete write, in their own words and in their own handwriting, a signed letter indicating their understanding of the risks of continued participation, and their willingness to assume these risks, instead of signing a waiver.[5,6] The difference is that a standard waiver is usually a form with blanks that are filled in by the physician and written in language that the parents or athlete would not normally use. With the standard waiver form, it has been successfully argued in court that, despite having signed a waiver, the parent and athlete did not fully understand the risks involved. However, with a letter written by the parents and/or athlete, it would be difficult to convince a jury that the parents or athlete did not understand the risks prior to any adverse event that might occur from continued participation.

Standardized approach. Physicians have been inconsistent with clearance recommendations when athletes seek to participate with medical conditions considered by some to pose a risk to the athlete. Recent news dispatches have chronicled the college-hopping of athletes who were barred for medical reasons, such as repeated concussions or hypertrophic cardiomyopathy, at 1 institution only to find playing time through transfer to a different institution and/or a different set of physicians. This inconsistency confuses athletes, coaches, parents, and administrators, since no clear eligibility protocols are accepted across the nation, and the athlete's medical condition may not be accurately depicted in the media.

It would be desirable to have the medical profession establish a standard approach to some of these controversial conditions to be used by all for PPE clearance decisions until an evidence-based assessment can be made for each athlete. However, it seems impractical that "standard" recommendations mostly based on anecdotal data and the opinions of experts will be universally upheld by individual physicians and institutions.

Ideally, institutions would not use exculpatory waivers and instead rely on the recommendations of medical personnel to determine clearance for participation. The process is best administered when the school or sponsoring agent acts in concert with the medical team to promote the safest participation plan for the athlete and stands behind the decision of the medical providers.

SEXUAL HARASSMENT CLAIMS

The issue of improper professional conduct during the PPE has surfaced on several occasions with allegations of sexual improprieties on the part of the physician.[7] Although most of these complaints have involved male-to-female interactions, there have been some recent complaints by male athletes against male physicians. The station-based group examination format may present the greatest risk of such claims, given the typical lack of previous relationship between the patient-athlete and the examiner (see "Legal Ramifications of the Exam Setting," below).

There is always risk of false accusations in any patient encounter when the door is closed and the physician is alone with a patient; a chaperone in the room is recommended when this is a concern. Furthermore, athletes may not expect to have a thorough examination, and portions of the PPE, although proper, can be perceived as improper, particularly when the genitalia are involved. Obviously, common sense should prevail, and the exam should be tailored to the history.

In every case, the physician should inform the athlete of the extent and purpose of the physical examination prior to performing it; provide an appropriate setting, including chaperones; and use discretion with comments or actions that may be misconstrued.

LEGAL RAMIFICATIONS OF THE EXAM SETTING

The exam setting will have some bearing on all aspects of the PPE. Physicians who evaluate and recommend sports participation after completing a PPE in the office always face liability issues as they would with any patient encounter. An exam and clearance recommendation completed by the athlete's personal physician continues the physician-patient relationship with access to an ongoing medical record. This method therefore leaves less room for error and misunderstanding and less risk for missed or intentionally omitted medical information compared with group exams.

Offering exam stations with physicians of both genders and allowing athletes to choose the examiner during a multiple-physician exam can also decrease the risk of perceived impropriety. Consistency in patient attire during the examination (eg, males in shorts and T-shirts and females in shorts and tank tops under a T-shirt with shirts removed in the privacy of the exam room) and in the examination routine (eg, deferring female breast and genital examinations) will decrease the risk of an athlete's comparing his or her examination with those of other athletes and questioning why it might have been different.

GOOD SAMARITAN STATUTES

The legal liability of those who perform PPEs on a volunteer basis is not easily understood. Good Samaritan statutes vary from state to state, and pro bono work is not always equated with Good Samaritan activities.[8] In some states, Good Samaritan statutes cover only those providers who step in to help in an emergency situation.

It is important for physicians to know their state's statutes regarding PPEs in the volunteer setting and, if they wish to be protected by a Good Samaritan statute, be aware that they cannot accept any form of remuneration for their services. A planned PPE at a school or clinic would not qualify as a Good Samaritan intervention under statutes that cover only emergency situations. Physicians who volunteer as examiners in mass screening PPE sessions that are not covered under a Good Samaritan statute must address the issue of malpractice insurance coverage during volunteer activities, especially outside the office and hospital setting. It is prudent for physicians to check with their insurance carrier before volunteering at PPE sessions or on the sidelines of a local game or meet.

HIPAA AND FERPA REGULATIONS

The Health Insurance Portability and Accountability Act (HIPAA), in 1996, and the Family Education Rights and Privacy Act (FERPA), in 1974, were developed, in part, to regulate "protected health information." "Protected health information" identifies an athlete relating to past, present, or future physical or mental health conditions. HIPAA regulations define protected health information as "any information, whether oral or recorded in any form or medium" that "is created or received by a healthcare provider, health plan, public health authority, employer, life insurer, school or university, or healthcare clearinghouse" and "relates to the past, present, or future physical or mental health or condition of an individual; the provision of healthcare to an individual; or the past, present, or future payment for the provision of healthcare to an individual."

HIPAA. HIPAA protects the privacy of health information through applicable federal privacy and confidentiality requirements in healthcare settings that use electronic billing. It was designed to create a single uniform and electronic system to check eligibility, record data, exchange information, and pay claims to reduce healthcare costs. At the same time, HIPAA created new and uniform federal standards for protecting the privacy of patient records.

The full impact of HIPAA is just now being felt by the healthcare profession. The US Department of Health and Human Services (HHS) has published HIPAA rules on everything from the categories used to record patient information to the security requirements and privacy rules for keeping patient records. HIPAA may not always apply to issues related to the PPE, but the culture of medical practice and patients' expectations will be set by the specter of the HIPAA statutes with respect to confidentiality, record security, and informed consent.

Contrary to HIPAA myth, its Privacy Rule expressly allows release of medical information without the individual's authorization for treatment, consulting with other providers, referring the patient to other providers, and notifying the patient's family. The "cleared" or "not cleared" decision relayed without other medical information falls within these categories and can be given to coaches and school administrators who need to know the player's medical eligibility.[9] A signed authorization for release of patient information must be obtained for any uses that fall outside of treatment and healthcare operation activities if the physician is not employed by the athlete's school or if the physician's billing transactions involve electronic transmission.

FERPA. Within the domain of the public schools, FERPA regulations prevail. FERPA regulations have similar intent and govern public school employees like school nurses, school physicians, coaches, and certified athletic trainers. Some states have interpreted the law to mean that a HIPAA authorization is not needed for release of information in the public school setting because FERPA prevails, but it may be prudent to incorporate HIPAA regulations despite these interpretations.

Any athlete who is seen in a medical facility outside the school will most likely fall within the purview of HIPAA. High school, college, and professional team physicians will be treated differently, and each physician should determine how he or she fits into the scheme of HIPAA and FERPA regulations.

Confidentiality with forms. For the purposes of participation clearance in a private practice setting, it would seem safest to separate the clearance form from the recorded confidential history and physical portions of the exam—as we do in this monograph. The alternative would be to have a clear release of medical information clause and appropriate athlete or parent signature that allows the information to go to the school or team. A copy of the history and physical exam form should stay with the athlete's medical record. With or without HIPAA and FERPA, athletes have a right to privacy, and all medical interactions should respect confidentiality.

For group exams, the issue of confidential storage of the forms must be addressed. The information pertaining to restrictions should be shared only with those in the school administration who need to know. A copy of the form should be made available to the athlete's primary physician, if possible and permitted by the athlete or parents.

The forms in this monograph reflect the restrictions placed on protected health information and are designed to share information with those essential to the process of athlete evaluation, emergency care, and future sports participation.

Who needs to know? Beyond the PPE, a return to participation after injury and illness requires similar attention to privacy and may require some form of release to discuss the issues with the team coaches and athletic trainers that go beyond clearance and treatment issues, respectively. The question that should guide the transfer of information is, "Who really needs to know?" In most team circumstances, the athletic trainer needs to know the medical details that apply to the athletic setting, and the coach and administration need to know only if the athlete is eligible to participate.

One suggested, but legally untested, strategy for compliance is to require that an authorization for

physicians, coaches, and athletic trainers to share necessary information for the good of the athlete be a requirement for participation in the school sports activity program. Once the information is into the domain of the school, FERPA regulations prevail. All coaches, administrators, certified athletic trainers, and schools should receive education on how to follow regulations on athlete privacy. Education for coaches and activities directors or athletic directors will help maintain privacy regulations. Sports organizations need to develop educational programs to ensure that all involved in the process are aware of the intent and legal constraints. For the purposes of athlete confidentiality and privacy regulations, all coaches, certified athletic trainers, and schools are expected to follow the guidelines.

Sharing emergency and public health information. For athlete safety and quick response to emergency situations, the clearance form should include, for sideline use, emergency information such as known allergies. The athletic trainer should have access to a listing of chronic medical problems and medications for emergency care when parents are not available. When an athletic trainer is not available, one of the coaching staff should have this information.

Even if consent is not obtained, some health information needs to be shared with athletic trainers and appropriate coaches when public health and safety may be at risk. For example, if an athlete develops an infectious disease such as herpes gladiatorum or meningococcal meningitis, the coach may notify an opposing team of potential contact during the infectious period of the disease. This may help prevent or reduce the transmission of the disease to others and is particularly important in sports with frequent and traumatic skin contact, like wrestling, where knowledge of a herpes skin infection would benefit past and future opponents. Privacy protection was not intended to interfere with public health.

Some situations require disclosure of health information to public health authorities, including but not limited to:

✦ Reporting reactions to medications or problems with products;

✦ Preventing or controlling disease, injury, or disability (similar to state and federal reportable disease lists);

✦ Notifying athletes of recalls of products they may be using; and

✦ Notifying athletes or coaches who may have been exposed to a disease or may be at risk of contracting or spreading a disease or condition.

Electronic transmission. When coaches and athletic trainers use electronic record systems to store and transport information needed to treat athletes, the information systems must be secure from access by unauthorized people. One example is that e-mail communications to and from a coach or athletic trainer may not be secure when sent through public communication lines like the Internet. Athletes need to give permission for physicians to communicate personal health information with coaches and athletic trainers via e-mail.

Restricting information. Athletes have the right to request a restriction or limitation on the health information the school uses or discloses. The request must be in writing to the facility where the team records are maintained (see appendix A on page 97 for an example of a consent form). The request must state (1) what information is to be limited; (2) whether the limit pertains to use, disclosure or both; and (3) to whom the limits apply. The athlete may also request that all confidential communications be conducted away from the practice sessions, games sites, and locker rooms. For those seeking more detail about HIPAA, the HHS Office of Civil Rights maintains a Web site at www.hhs.gov/ocr/hipaa that provides a variety of helpful information, including forms and many educational materials about the Privacy Rule.

When traveling. Ideally, the information obtained during the PPE should be available to the team physician, team athletic trainer, and emergency medical personnel, who may all be called to render emergency care for an athlete on the sideline or in the training room. Many teams travel with a copy of the PPE medical form in case the athlete is injured during an away game. When the team physician does the PPE and keeps a secured copy of the exam form for use in these situations, the solution to the problem of confidentiality and the PPE record is simplified.

When athletes in high schools have exams completed by their primary physicians, however, confidentiality is a bit more complicated. A history of diabetes, seizures, asthma, or allergies can be critical in certain instances. The clearance form developed for this monograph attempts to address this issue by including allergies and other emergency information. In addi-

tion, it falls to the athlete and/or parents to inform the on-site physician, athletic trainer, or coach of medical conditions that might result in an emergency for the athlete.

◥ COMPETITIONS FOR THE PHYSICALLY OR COGNITIVELY IMPAIRED

Several states have physically impaired (PI) and cognitively impaired (CI) competition groupings at the high school level. The criteria for inclusion in these groups are defined by each state. The fairness of the competitions requires that the qualification criteria are strictly defined and enforced, because individuals who are more qualified than the inclusion criteria allow upset the balance of competition and increase the risk of injury to the other competitors.

Physically impaired. PI competition criteria require that there is an actual physical defect that limits participation in regular competition, such as a neuromuscular, postural or skeletal, traumatic, growth, or neurologic impairment or loss of limb that significantly impairs physical functioning, modifies gait patterns, or requires mobility devices. PI competition is not for those who do not qualify for CI competition or cannot make the cut for regular competition without some form of physical limitation. In Minnesota, high school PI competition specifically excludes asthma, diabetes mellitus, seizure disorder, attention deficit disorder, Tourette's syndrome, autistic spectrum disorders, deafness, blindness, obesity, and similar maladies that may interfere with regular competition but do not involve an actual physical impairment.

Cognitively impaired. CI competition is for individuals with lower IQ levels, commonly less than 70. A physical handicap is not a prerequisite for CI competition, and participants with higher IQ levels than the prescribed cutoff could dominate the events. These athletes enjoy the competition and social nature of the events and deserve to participate on a "level playing field" with others of similar cognitive ability.

Special Olympics and Paralympics. In the community setting, athletes participate in Special Olympic and Paralympic competitions. Each organization has its own set of governing rules and inclusion criteria for competition.

Paralympics assigns numerical rank to the level of disability. Teams need to stay within a defined sum of the grades to compete. If a 2-person sailboat can have a team total of 8; a 2 can pair with a 6, a 3 can pair with a 5, and a 4 can pair with a 4. Again, this arrangement provides fair participation. Accurate assessment of ability, of course, is critical to the competition.

Special Olympics has requirements for PPE assessment that include radiographic imaging for atlantoaxial instability in asymptomatic trisomy 21 competitors. Further rules and regulations for Paralympic and Special Olympics competitions with respect to the PPE are discussed in detail in "The Athlete With Special Needs," chapter 8 (page 79).

REFERENCES

1. Gallup EM: Law and the Team Physician. Champaign, IL, Human Kinetics 1995, pp 77, 80-81
2. Maron BJ, Mitten MJ, Quandt EF, et al: Competitive athletes with cardiovascular disease: the case of Nicholas Knapp. N Engl J Med 1998;339(22):1632-1635
3. Gallup EM: Law and the Team Physician. Champaign, IL, Human Kinetics, 1995, p 45
4. Herbert DL: Prospective releases: will their use protect sports medicine physicians from suit? Sports Med Stand Malpract Rep 1994;6(3):33, 35-36
5. Jones CJ: College athletes: illness or injury and the decision to return to play. Buffalo Law Rev 1992;40:113-215
6. Mitten MJ: Team physicians and competitive athletes: allocating legal responsibilities for athletic injuries. U Pitt Law Rev 1993;55:129-169
7. Herbert DL: Professional considerations related to the conduct of preparticipation examinations. Sports Med Stand Malpract Rep 1994;6(4):49, 51-52
8. Gallup EM: Law and the Team Physician. Champaign, IL, Human Kinetics, 1995, pp 76-77
9. Magee JT, Almekinders LC, Taft TN: HIPAA and the team physician. Sports Med Update 2003;March-April:4-7

Chapter 5

The PPE Medical History

The medical history is the most crucial component of the preparticipation evaluation. A complete history will identify approximately 75% of problems affecting athletes.[1,2] With approximately 4 million competitive athletes in high school alone[3] and 30 million under age 18 who play on some sort of organized sports team in the United States,[4] there are great challenges to devising a screening tool that will be thorough and user-friendly. The questions developed for the medical history portion of the PPE are designed to screen for conditions that would place the athlete at unacceptable medical risk, understanding that it is not possible to achieve a zero-risk circumstance in competitive sports.[5]

The most accurate and detailed information is obtained when athletes and parents or guardians complete the history form together before the evaluation. In a comparison study,[1] only 39% of the athletes' responses agreed with information given by the parents completing the same form. Illiteracy or language barriers may further diminish the accuracy of responses to the medical history questions. In athletes for whom English is a second language, assistance may be required. Ideally, a physician will review the history in a private setting with the athlete prior to the PPE physical examination. Any abnormalities found on the history form should elicit further history for explanation.

The AAP states that children should have a medical "home" and should know the name of their physician.[6] Often, they do not. The PPE may be the only time athletes meet with a physician. It may be the only opportunity they have to receive a medical screening and discuss their concerns. The PPE is fully utilized when information about health, risks to health, and identification of conditions that may influence athletic performance is obtained. It is our view that the PPE should not be focused solely on "clearance" for participation, but rather a "qualification" for appropriate activity and an opportunity to influence safe and healthy lifestyle decisions.

We have reviewed the literature on PPEs, including numerous forms used nationwide, in the preparation of this monograph. As expected, there are more similarities than differences. We endeavor to provide a comprehensive form that is clinically relevant and easily used by busy athletes, parents, and physicians. This chapter details the rationale for the "primary questions," or those listed on the PPE history form (page 93). It also offers suggestions for "secondary," or follow-up, questions for "yes" responses to primary questions. References are included for scientific integrity and to encourage further inquiry into the reasoning behind the exam and process.

Primary questions on the PPE form address fundamental issues of greatest concern for sports participation and general health risk during physical activity. Background information and rationale for the inclusion of the primary questions are available in this monograph. Where possible, we have used validated questions from sources such as the Youth Risk Behavior Surveillance System (YRBSS).[7] Adoption of a widely used and standardized PPE form can help create a database that can shape future health policy and research directions.

Secondary questions serve as a guide for physicians to gather more in-depth information that may affect the athlete's health and safety. Secondary questions appear in boxes within the text but not on the form.

A "Teen Screen," (appendix B, page 98), is designed to guide the examiner regarding inquiries into high-risk behaviors and is not intended to be included on the PPE form. In addition, the physical examination form (page 94) includes questions to be pursued by the physician on high-risk behaviors, and not to be filled in by the patient. These issues are discussed at the end of this chapter (page 36).

What the PPE should cover is the subject of much debate. There are those who would strictly limit the assessment to a cardiovascular and musculoskeletal examination only. Others advocate for a broader assessment to include prevention strategies and inquiry about high-risk behavior. Because it would prove difficult to glean truthful information to written questions on such sensitive topics, we have opted for obtaining the information via direct physician questioning, as just mentioned.

Finally, medical technology and increased general awareness of the multiple benefits of athletics have broadened opportunities for participation to groups that have traditionally been overlooked. More than 54 million Americans have physical disabilities, and there are expanded opportunities available to those who aspire to compete but who are physically or intellectually disabled. (See "The Athlete With Special Needs," chapter 8, page 79.) Physicians evaluating Special Olympians and Paralympians can use this monograph for their PPE, as we have created a form that we hope can be used by all young athletes.

◣ MEDICAL HISTORY

1. Has a doctor ever denied or restricted your participation in sports for any reason?

2. Do you have an ongoing medical condition (like diabetes or asthma)?

Prior denial or restriction to participation is a significant finding that requires investigation. Only approximately 1% to 2% of screened athletes are completely disqualified from sports participation,[8,9] so to have been denied clearance is noteworthy. In-depth assessment is warranted to determine if the disqualifying condition is still present or has been treated. If the condition is still present, the physician and athlete should discuss issues that will affect safe play, including risks of participation, the use of assistive devices, and alternative sports that may better fit the physical or mental challenges of the athlete.

This may be more in-depth than time permits during a standard PPE. If so, a follow-up appointment or referral to a specialist is recommended. If the condition has been treated, determination should be made about the extent of recovery and clearance for participation.

Chronic medical conditions must be noted to determine the basic health status of the athlete. This is an opportunity for the physician to get a "big picture" of the athlete's general health. Such questions can be a springboard for further inquiries and discussions. Chronic medical conditions may affect performance and clearance. Inadequate control of conditions such as asthma, seizures, or even skin disease may affect the ability to play. An athlete who requires frequent hospital admissions for diabetes, seizures, or acute asthma would likely need further medical evaluation before competing. Use of certain medications for common conditions may affect performance or safety and may even be banned, depending on the sport. Some medications may affect judgment, reflexes, or stamina.

Athletes should be counseled about the impact of their medical condition on performance even if they are fully cleared for participation.

SECONDARY QUESTIONS
+ **When and why were you disqualified from participation?**
+ **Have you seen a doctor for this condition?**
+ **What has changed since you were disqualified?**

◣ MEDICATIONS AND SUPPLEMENTS

3. Are you currently taking any prescription or nonprescription (over-the-counter) medicines or pills?

Medications—prescription or nonprescription—taken by athletes may reveal medical problems that the athlete may have omitted in the queries about medical history. Many over-the-counter medications and supplements, herbs, or minerals are not considered important or of consequence by athletes or their parents or guardians. The PPE setting can be used as an opportunity to discuss and counsel athletes and parents about the risks of medications, supplements, and ergogenic aids.

In every medical encounter, truthfulness is required for optimal care, and we acknowledge that some athletes may not be forthcoming with information about medication or supplements. However, it is important to inquire and to invite conversation and counseling about substances the athlete may be taking.

Some over-the-counter medications can affect performance and may even be banned by the sport's national governing body (NGB). For example, antihistamines may cause fatigue and light-headedness. Arrhythmias have been linked to beta-agonists, methylxanthines, tricyclic antidepressants, decongestants, and macrolide antibiotics. Fluoroquinolone antibiotics have been shown to increase the risk of tendinitis, tendon degeneration, and tendon rupture.[10,11] Supplements are discussed in more detail later in this monograph.

SECONDARY QUESTION
+ Do you take herbs or minerals?

◼ ALLERGIES AND ANAPHYLAXIS

4. Do you have allergies to medicines, pollens, foods, or stinging insects?

Allergic reactions range from minor rhinitis to anaphylaxis. Outdoor environments potentially expose the athlete to stinging insects and allergens. Allergy to hymenoptera (eg, bee, wasp, yellow jacket, and fire ant) envenomation and/or a history of exercise-induced anaphylaxis or exercise-induced urticaria should be noted. Aggressive inquiry into details of past events should be documented so that severity of reaction can be determined, and, in the case of anaphylactic reaction, appropriate treatments can be available for practice and competition.

Cholinergic urticaria is an exaggerated cholinergic response to body warming. Urticarial papules may first appear on the upper thorax and neck and then spread to the entire body after exposure to heat and humidity.[12] Individual lesions usually persist for 15 to 20 minutes, but continued reaction and the development of new lesions may affect the athlete for several hours.[12] This phenomenon is a histamine-mediated reaction that rarely results in vascular collapse.

Anaphylaxis refers to symptoms involving more than 1 body system and can start as localized erythema and edema, followed by generalized urticaria and pruritus and even laryngeal edema and spasm leading to airway obstruction. Insect stings or food allergies—especially to shellfish or peanuts—can lead to anaphylaxis. Food sensitivities can also limit calorie sources and affect energy balance in athletes.

Exercise-induced anaphylaxis is a rare form of physical allergy that is induced by exercise and is characterized by a spectrum of symptoms, from a sensation of warmth, pruritus, cutaneous erythema, angioedema, and giant urticaria (more than 1 cm), to hypotension, shock, and death.[12] The role of exercise in eliciting symptoms remains obscure. Dependent factors include a variety of specific foods (eg, wheat, mushrooms, grapes, wine, onions, snails, corn, garlic, milk, or eggs). There are two types of exercise-induced anaphylaxis: classic and variant.[12] These immunoglobulin E–mediated responses can result in bronchospasm, pulmonary distress, hemodynamic instability, and even shock.

Athletes who are most at risk for serious reaction should be required to have injectable epinephrine (eg, EpiPen) on site for immediate use. Coaches and medical staff should be aware of the athlete's predisposition to anaphylaxis and be trained and prepared to intervene.

SECONDARY QUESTIONS
- Were you hospitalized?
- Were you intubated?
- Do you carry an EpiPen?

◼ CARDIOVASCULAR PROBLEMS

5. Have you ever passed out or nearly passed out DURING exercise?

6. Have you ever passed out or nearly passed out AFTER exercise?

7. Have you ever had discomfort, pain, or pressure in your chest during exercise?

8. Does your heart race or skip beats during exercise?

9. Has a doctor ever told you that you have high blood pressure, high cholesterol, a heart murmur, or a heart infection?

10. Has a doctor ever ordered a test for your heart (for example, ECG, echocardiogram)?

11. Has anyone in your family died for no apparent reason?

12. Does anyone in your family have a heart problem?

13. Has any family member or relative died of heart problems or of sudden death before age 50?

14. Does anyone in your family have Marfan syndrome?

The detection of potentially life-threatening conditions is one of the goals of the PPE, but detecting potentially life-threatening cardiovascular conditions in asymptomatic athletes at the PPE is exceedingly difficult. Most often, the first sign of a cardiac abnormality is sudden death.

The AHA states that the purpose of screening is to provide medical clearance for participation in competitive sports through routine and systematic evaluations intended to identify clinically relevant and preexisting cardiovascular abnormalities and thereby reduce the risks associated with organized sports.[3] The AHA recommends that some form of preparticipation cardiovascular screening for high school and collegiate athletes is justifiable and compelling, based on ethical, legal, and medical grounds.[3] Any previous disqualification from athletics because of a cardiac condition should be thoroughly investigated before a clearance decision is made. The 26th Bethesda Conference provides information about guidelines for clearance of athletes who have a cardiac condition.[13]

Life-threatening cardiac conditions are rare, and detecting them during a large-scale standard PPE presents significant challenges.[3] Only about 20% are diagnosed before sudden death.[14] It is unrealistic on the part of physicians and the general public to expect that the PPE can exclude most of the important cardiac lesions.[14]

Sudden death occurs in the range of 1:100,000 to 1:300,000 high school-age athletes and is disproportionately higher in males.[14,15] Structural cardiac problems leading to fatal arrhythmias account for more than 95% of sudden deaths in athletes under age 30.[16-19] Sudden cardiac death in young athletes was reported to be caused by a primary cardiac disorder in 85% of cases.[14] Of these, 36% had hypertrophic cardiomyopathy and 13% had anomalous coronary arteries.[14] Basketball, American football, track, and soccer have the highest incidence of sudden death in young athletes.[3]

Among athletes of all ages, more experience sudden cardiac death from coronary artery disease than from other causes.[5,20] However, when cardiac abnormalities are detected or suspected, the AHA recommends referral to a cardiovascular specialist.

The primary questions were developed after scrutiny of the literature and are meant to elicit responses that may hint of the presence of serious cardiac conditions and lead to further investigation. Secondary questions should include symptoms of exercise intolerance, onset and duration of symptoms, caffeine consumption, and supplement and medication use.

Syncope (complete loss of consciousness) or **near syncope** (dizziness or light-headedness) may be an indicator of autonomic instability (vasovagal syncope), bradyarrhythmias, or tachyarrhythmias, which are rare in athletes.[21] Nonarrhythmic cardiac conditions causing syncope include aortic stenosis (eg, hypertrophic cardiomyopathy) or mitral valve prolapse. Noncardiac causes include hypoglycemia, migraines, and medications.

Syncope or near syncope during exercise may herald a more serious, and likely, cardiac disorder. Athletes with this history should be screened for potentially lethal conditions.[18] Among athletes experiencing sudden death, syncope was associated in 17% of cases in 1 study[14] and 23% in another.[22] This history warrants detailed family and personal history of cardiac disease and personal use of medications and illicit drug use.[23]

Syncope or near syncope after exercise is much less ominous than during exercise and more likely to be secondary to hypotension. An example is exercise-associated collapse commonly observed at endurance events. Nonetheless, such a history deserves follow-up inquiry and possible workup to exclude the presence of a cardiac or other serious condition.

Chest discomfort, pain, or pressure in young athletes is a common presenting complaint and one for which true cardiac disease is uncommon.[18,24-26] Chest pain on exertion may indicate advanced atherosclerotic disease (unusual before age 30 except with abnormal lipid metabolism) or congenital abnormalities of the coronary arteries. Adolescents may describe "chest pain," "chest discomfort," "heart racing," or "chest flutters" in describing sensation associated with arrhythmias. However, in the pediatric population, chest pain is more commonly from exercise-induced asthma (EIA) than from a cardiac source.[25] An athlete who has chest discomfort, pain, or pressure during exercise with other symptoms such as syncope or presyncope should be evaluated for a cardiac disorder.[18]

Dyspnea on exertion may indicate structural abnormalities; valve problems; underlying pulmonary disease, especially EIA; or poor conditioning. Palpitations or skipped beats may signify arrhythmias or conduction abnormalities, such as Wolff-Parkinson-White syndrome. Such symptoms may mandate further investigation before clearance.

Heart "racing" or "skipping beats," palpitations, or other abnormal sensation of heart beating are indicative of arrhythmias.[21] Palpitations may be irregular or regular and may be associated with presyncope or syncope. A detailed history will elicit information to determine whether the palpitations are significant or require further investigation. If they are associated with symptoms of exercise intolerance such as light-headedness, dizziness, or chest discomfort, cardiac disease should be investigated.

Hypertension is the most common cardiovascular condition seen in people who engage in competitive athletics.[27] There has been a general trend of increasing body size among athletes, which may falsely lead to labeling an athlete as being hypertensive. Elevated blood pressure was reported in 6.4% of athletes presenting for routine PPE.[28] Repeat blood pressure monitoring and use of pediatric hypertensive guidelines (see the cardiovascular section of "Determining Clearance," page 67), which correlate age, blood pressure, and height percentile from growth charts, is recommended.[18,29,30] Recommendations for follow-up, counseling on healthy lifestyles behaviors, and determination of eligibility for competition should be made.[31]

Hypercholesterolemia and hyperlipidemia are associated with coronary artery disease and sudden cardiac death. Inquiry during the personal history should invite opportunity for query into the history of management strategies and most recent testing. These conditions in the presence of symptoms of exercise intolerance should warrant further investigation. In the face of increasing incidence of childhood obesity and type 2 diabetes mellitus, the AAP and American Diabetic Association have issued guidelines regarding screening of children for dyslipidemia.[32,33]

Murmurs that are "innocent" are estimated to occur in up to 50% of children,[34-36] with approximately 5% having significant, or "guilty," murmurs. Innocent murmurs are typically grade 1 or 2 and manifest early and as the midsystolic vibratory or musical-type (Still's) murmur. Frequently, these athletes have been told that they have a murmur, and no workup was performed. In the absence of symptoms of exercise intolerance, an "innocent" murmur requires no further investigation. If doubt persists, even after thorough history and auscultatory examination, referral for a 2-D/Doppler echocardiogram or referral to a cardiovascular specialist is recommended.

Significant murmurs indicate underlying heart disease. They are typically loud (usually grade 3 or more) and may be holosystolic, late systolic, systolic ejection with or without a click, diastolic, or continuous. Systolic ejection or midsystolic clicks typically are abnormal at any age and usually imply an abnormal cardiac status.[18,37]

Heart infections include myocarditis, endocarditis, and pericarditis. Myocarditis most often is viral in origin and may cause minimal symptoms such as tachycardia, fatigue, and mild abdominal or chest distress.[18] More serious symptoms, such as congestive heart failure, tachypnea, tachycardia, or hepatomegaly, may be present.[37,38] A history of recent viral symptoms or acute illness usually can be elicited.

Heart tests such as ECG, echocardiogram, and exercise treadmill testing performed previously on the athlete may indicate a history of cardiac disorder or suspected disorder that the athlete had not previous revealed, likely through benign forgetfulness. This history is important and should be investigated fully. Obtaining medical records describing the specific tests and their results can be very beneficial. The athlete's recall as to why the tests were ordered and whether circumstances warranting prior workup still persist is critical.

Sudden unexplained death, especially in a first- or second-degree relative before age 50, may indicate that the athlete is at greater risk of sudden cardiac death (table 4).[39,40] Because the death is "unexplained," it cannot be known with certainty that the cause was cardiac. However, it must be presumed that the cause was sudden cardiac death. The athlete and parent or guardian should be asked about the circumstances of the death and the prior health or symptoms of the deceased relative. An athlete with this history should be considered for basic workup, including ECG, echocardiogram, and lipid panel (table 5).

Family history of heart disease may confer a greater risk of heart disease in the athlete. Because several causes of sudden cardiac death may be familial (for example, hypertrophic cardiomyopathy, Marfan syndrome, and lipid abnormalities causing coronary artery disease), inquiring about family cardiac history is important. Examiners should query to determine if high-risk factors such as diabetes, hypertension, or an abnormal lipid profile are present in the family. Arrhythmias such as long QT syndrome and conditions such as Marfan syndrome and Ehlers-Danlos syndrome can be familial and confer greater risk of arrhythmia to the athlete.

Family history of sudden death before age 50 is significant, because it indicates that the cause, absent trauma, was, most likely, cardiac related. For the athlete, this means a greater personal risk for sudden death (see table 4). At the PPE, a plan should be made for more extensive evaluation (see table 5), including a more detailed medical history and possible ECG and laboratory investigation, to assess the athlete for a heart condition.

| **Table 4** | **Conditions Causing Increased Risk for Sudden Cardiac Death in Young Athletes** |

Hypertrophic cardiomyopathy
Long QT syndrome
  Congenital
  Acquired
Marfan syndrome
Ehlers-Danlos syndrome
Arrhythmogenic right ventricular
  cardiomyopathy
Commotio cordis
Dilated cardiomyopathy
Acquired cardiac disease
  Myocardial
  Pericardial
  Endocardial
Congenital heart disease
  Aortic stenosis
  Coarctation of aorta

Mitral valve prolapse
Anomalous coronary arteries
Postoperative congenital heart arrhythmias
  Postoperative tetralogy of Fallot
  Postoperative atrial switch transposition of
    great vessels
  Postoperative atrial septal defect repair
Brugada syndrome
Wolff-Parkinson-White syndrome (pre-excitation syndrome)
Congenital heart block
  Möbitz type 2
  Third-degree (complete) heart block

Reprinted with permission from Luckstead EF: Cardiac risk factors and participation guidelines for youth sports. Pediatr Clin North Am 2002;49(4):681-707.

| **Table 5** | **Noninvasive Cardiac Screening Tests** |

Test	Good for Detecting
ECG	Long QT interval Pre-excitation syndrome Bundle branch block Abnormal Q waves with T-wave changes Cardiac hypertrophy Dysrhythmias
Echocardiography	Hypertrophic cardiomyopathy Valvular abnormalities Aortic root dilatation Left ventricular dysfunction Myopericardial conditions
Exercise stress testing	Coronary artery disease Long QT syndrome Exercise-induced tachyarrythmias
Electrophysiologic study	Conduction abnormalities
Chest radiography	Cardiac enlargement Increased pulmonary vascularity

ECG = electrocardiography

Marfan syndrome is an inherited connective-tissue disease that is autosomal dominant and manifests clinically with characteristic physical findings (table 6). Genetic disorders like Marfan syndrome do not always manifest with the classic phenotype, and therefore a family history of the disorder should trigger an investigation. Aortic root dilatation, common in Marfan syndrome, can lead to aortic dissection and rupture and sudden death. Screening of athletes is recommended for men taller than 6 ft and women taller than 5 ft, 10 in., who have 2 or more physical manifestations or a family history of Marfan syndrome.[41] Investigation should include ECG, slit-lamp eye examination, and echocardiogram to assess the aortic root.

Table 6	**Physical Stigmata of Marfan Syndrome**

Kyphosis
High-arched palate
Pectus excavatum
Arachnodactyly
Arm span > height
Mitral valve prolapse
Aortic insufficiency (murmur)
Myopia
Lenticular dislocation
'Thumb sign'
'Wrist sign'

SECONDARY QUESTIONS

◆ Have you ever been to a doctor for this?
◆ What tests have you had?
◆ Have you missed any practices or games because of this?
◆ What symptoms have you had when you exercise?
◆ When do symptoms begin, and how long do they last?
◆ Do you take caffeine, supplements, or medication?

◼ SURGICAL HISTORY

15. Have you ever spent the night in a hospital?
16. Have you ever had surgery?

Surgical history or hospitalization is significant and may potentially affect clearance determinations or guide conditioning or rehabilitation programs. The surgeon must clear an athlete who has had recent surgery. For surgeries, such as appendectomy or tonsillectomy, there would be reasonable expectation for full recovery with no long-term impact on athletic participation or performance. Other surgeries, such as colon resection with colostomy or those that remove 1 of a paired set of organs, such as enucleation, may affect clearance or performance and require counseling about risks of further injury and also about protective equipment.

Athletes with illnesses for which surgery and chronic use of medication are aspects of treatment should be advised about the potential impact of medications on athletic performance. For example, where there is no formal drug testing program, such as with most club sports and high schools, the use of narcotics, although not banned, may impair thought processes, reflexes, and stamina.

Orthopedic surgery requires successful postopera-

tive recovery and, in some cases, many months of rehabilitation for successful return to full participation. At the PPE, the athlete should be asked not only about the type of surgery but also the type and duration of the rehabilitation program (eg, physical therapy, home rehab program, or none). Operative repair of a joint injury, even years previously, without adequate rehabilitation, can leave the joint weakened and susceptible to further injury. Query should also be made about the use of braces or taping.

SECONDARY QUESTIONS

◆ What surgery did you have?
◆ When did you have it?
◆ Where did you have it?
◆ Do you still have problems from your surgery?
◆ Did you do rehabilitation or see a physical therapist?

◼ MUSCULOSKELETAL INJURY

17. Have you ever had an injury, like a sprain, muscle or ligament tear, or tendinitis, that caused you to miss a practice or game?
18. Have you had any broken or fractured bones or dislocated joints?
19. Have you ever had a stress fracture?
20. Have you had a bone or joint injury that required x-rays, MRI, CT, surgery, injections, rehabilitation, physical therapy, a brace, a cast, or crutches?
21. Have you been told that you have or have you had an x-ray for atlantoaxial (neck) instability?
22. Do you regularly use a brace or assistive device?

Musculoskeletal injuries are very common in sports and should be reviewed at the PPE. Most athletes at some point in their careers have experienced muscle, bone, or joint injury. Most often, these do not lead to chronic conditions or have long-term adverse effects on athletic participation. The primary questions listed here are designed to elicit responses regarding more serious injuries that may have long-term adverse effects on participation. Athletes should be assessed for physical limitations as a result of musculoskeletal injury so that further injury may be prevented through rehabilitation or bracing.

Missed practices or games or the use of braces or other devices may also be an indicator of the seriousness of the injury or condition. In such cases, inquiry should be made regarding mechanism of injury and prior medical or operative care. Documentation should include any specific rehabilitation program provided, including type and duration of exercise therapy and physical modalities. The physician should determine whether the athlete was declared fully rehabilitated by the treating physician or physical therapist and what recommendations were given to maintain strength and flexibility. In athletes with unresolved musculoskeletal pain, further workup may be warranted to exclude conditions such as occult fracture, tendinopathy, or rheumatologic disorders.

Fractures or dislocated joints are more serious orthopedic injuries. Detailed information about mechanism of injury, sport involved, treatment, and rehabilitation history should be obtained. Dislocated joints are frequently accompanied by a fracture. Such a major injury can confer permanent neurologic deficits. In such cases, referral to an orthopedic surgeon, physiatrist, neurologist, or other specialist for advice on clearance should be considered. Athletes should be asked about the use of braces, taping, or assistive devices.

Stress fractures are commonly observed in running sports and sports for which judging is subjective and appearance is important (eg, figure skating, gymnastics).[42,43] Osteoporosis and osteopenia from inadequate caloric intake can lead to stress fractures. An athlete with a history of stress fractures should be queried about disordered eating and inadequate caloric and calcium intake. Females should be asked about menstrual history, because inadequate caloric intake and body mass index (BMI) less than 18 kg/m^2 (underweight) may indicate disordered eating or the female athlete triad of disordered eating, osteoporosis or osteopenia, and amenorrhea.

Overtraining is a major cause of stress fractures.[43,44] Type of training schedule at the time of the stress fracture and modifications of training should be determined at the PPE. The type of shoe worn by athletes can contribute to lower-extremity stress fractures. Shoes designed for the athlete's specific sport such as volleyball, basketball, or cross-country should be encouraged. Examination for conditions that affect normal biomechanics of the lower extremity such as pes planus, pes cavus, or

overpronation should be made so that corrective devices such as orthoses be considered.

A history of x-rays, magnetic resonance imaging (MRI), computed tomography (CT), surgery, injections, rehabilitation, physical therapy, bracing, casting, or crutch use gives the physician a better idea of whether a previous injury has been serious. We have attempted to prompt athletes into remembering a procedure or workup, even if they may have forgotten the injury when answering previous questions. Such a history may provide valuable information when assessing the current status of the athlete.

Atlantoaxial instability (AAI) is common in athletes with Down syndrome. It is estimated that about 15% of children with Down syndrome have AAI,[45-47] almost all of whom are asymptomatic. Patients who have rheumatoid arthritis also have an increased risk of developing AAI. Children with skeletal dysplasias often have associated cervical spine instability with serious danger of spinal cord compression.[48]

General screening must include a history and physical examination, including neurologic assessment. Radiographic screening (generally lateral cervical spine with flexion and extension views) for AAI in asymptomatic athletes is controversial, because there is little evidence to suggest it is a significant risk factor for symptomatic AAI, a very rare condition in individuals with Down syndrome.[47] The condition appears as a space larger than 5 mm between the posterior aspect of the anterior arch of the atlas and the odontoid. Neurologic signs and symptoms (table 7)[47] may be more predictive of risk of injury progression than are radiographic abnormalities in asymptomatic patients.

Special Olympics mandates that all athletes with Down syndrome have preparticipation radiographic screening.[49] Those with AAI are not allowed to participate in activities that place the neck in extension, in-

Table 7	**Common Signs and Symptoms of Symptomatic Atlantoaxial Instability**
Easy fatigability	Sensory deficits
Difficulty in walking	Spasticity
Abnormal gait	Hyperreflexia
Neck pain	Clonus
Limited neck mobility	Extensor-plantar reflex
Torticollis	Upper motor neuron signs and symptoms
Incoordination and clumsiness	Posterior column signs and symptoms

cluding diving, the butterfly stroke and diving starts in swimming, gymnastics, the high jump, pentathlon, soccer, and any warm-up exercises that place pressure on the head and neck muscles. The AAP previously had a similar recommendation but dropped it, citing lack of evidence that asymptomatic AAI is a significant risk factor for symptomatic instability or dislocation.[50]

Atlantoaxial dislocation is rarer than AAI and confers greater risk to the athlete. Signs and symptoms are those of cord compression: abnormal gait, neck pain, limited neck mobility, head tilt, incoordination, clumsiness, and changes in bowel and bladder control. A neurologic examination may reveal sensory deficits, spasticity, hyperreflexia, clonus, and the presence of a Babinski sign.

Braces or other assistive devices used regularly provide insight into the functional capacity of the athlete. Types of knee braces include knee sleeves, postoperative, prophylactic, and functional. Frequently, athletes buy over-the-counter braces for relatively minor injuries sustained years previously, the utility of which should be discussed at the PPE. There is insufficient evidence that use of prophylactic knee braces prevents injury.[51]

Athletes with a history of surgery or permanent joint disability may use braces to counter the functional disability. Braces should be reevaluated prior to each season, as changes in body habitus may alter the fit of the brace and require modification to ensure proper fit and therefore proper protection of the joint.

ASTHMA

23. Has a doctor ever told you that you have asthma or allergies?

24. Do you cough, wheeze, or have difficulty breathing during or after exercise?

25. Is there anyone in your family who has asthma?

26. Have you ever used an inhaler or taken asthma medicine?

Asthma is a disease of inflammation of the airways characterized by airway hyperreactivity.[52] In susceptible individuals, this inflammation causes recurrent episodes of wheezing, breathlessness, chest tightness, and cough, particularly at night and in the early morning. These episodes are usually associated with widespread but variable airflow obstruction that is often reversible either spontaneously or with treatment. Inflammation also causes an associated increase in the existing bronchial hyperresponsiveness to a variety of stimuli. This in-

cludes, for some, exercise, such as running or playing hard, especially in cold weather, low humidity, or smoggy conditions. One child in 15 has asthma, according to the National Asthma Education and Prevention Program (NAEPP).[53]

Exercise-induced asthma has a prevalence in adolescents of 10% to 50%.[54-56] It can have significant impact on performance, frequently causing the athlete to have decreased stamina or to leave a practice or game. The disorder may be an isolated condition or be associated with intermittent or persistent asthma. Physicians must be aware that the history and symptoms alone fail to accurately identify persons with asthma or EIA 45.8% of the time.[53] The athlete may present with subtle symptoms, such as headaches, abdominal pains, muscle cramps, fatigue, dizziness, or "feeling out of shape."[52] The primary questions are intended to raise suspicion and invite further query. Recognition of EIA before sports participation may allow for the initiation of safe and effective preventive therapy and monitoring for worsening asthma.[53]

EIA may be diagnosed by maintaining a high index of suspicion (affirmative answers to primary questions) and by using peak expiratory flow rate measurements after exercise (table 8).[53,57,58] A detailed allergy and asthma history questionnaire was developed by the Sports Medicine Committee of the American College of Asthma, Allergy & Immunology[57] to assist in raising awareness of EIA. The primary questions above were developed to elicit responses suggestive of EIA.

For some athletes, spirometric testing may not provide clear evidence of obstruction, even in the face of true EIA. There is a segment of athletes with EIA who will falsely test negative unless testing is performed in the actual exercise setting or a similar setting. This is especially true for athletes whose symptoms are triggered by cold weather and whose testing is performed indoors. Testing in the sport environment or with the use of a methacholine challenge may aid in confirming the diagnosis. Exercise provokes symptoms in most children with previously diagnosed, poorly controlled asthma.

The physician should use the primary questions to discern whether there is a high likelihood of EIA and proceed with follow-up evaluation. Keep in mind that an affirmative answer to the previous question about chest discomfort (question #7) is more likely asthma than a cardiac condition. Inquiry must also be made into whether the athlete has a regular physician to help

Table 8	Spirometric Parameters for Diagnosing Asthma and Establishing Reversibility After Pharmacotherapy

Asthma Diagnosis
FEV_1 < 80% predicted
FEV_1/FVC < 65% or below the lower limit of normal

Establishing Reversibility After Short-Acting Inhaled Beta-2 Agonist
FEV_1 increases > 12% and ≥ 200 mL

FEV_1 = forced expiratory volume in 1 sec; FVC = forced vital capacity

manage the asthma and whether the athlete has medications for this condition.

Initiation of prophylactic measures may help athletes maximize their performance potential. Athletes with EIA often benefit from using their short-acting beta-agonist inhaler at least 5 to 10 minutes before exercise.[53] Long-acting beta agonists and leukotriene inhibitors are also effective in treating EIA, especially those athletes engaged in all-day activities like tournaments. They can be used 1 hour before activity. Antihistamines help control EIA in athletes for whom environmental allergens are a trigger; however, they may make the athlete feel fatigued. The NAEPP recommends that athletes warm up prior to practice or competition to help prevent or lessen episodes of EIA.[53] Athletes with asthma and a peak expiratory flow lower than 80% of their personal best should avoid running and vigorous play until the peak flow reading returns to at least 80% of their personal best.

The NAEPP recommends that a written asthma management plan be prepared for the athlete's school and should include plans to ensure reliable, prompt access to medications. Athletes with intermittent, persistent, or exercise-induced asthma should be required to have a short-acting beta-agonist metered dose inhaler on the sidelines of all practices and games. Athletes and coaches should be counseled that rescue medications must not be in the locker room but, rather, readily available.

SECONDARY QUESTIONS

◆ Where do you keep your inhaler/puffer?
◆ Have you ever missed practice or games because of your asthma?
◆ Have you gone to the hospital because of asthma during the past year?
◆ Have you ever been intubated?
◆ Who is the doctor for your asthma?

◤ PAIRED ORGANS

27. Were you born without or are you missing a kidney, an eye, a testicle, or any other organ?

The absence of one of a paired set of organs must be determined at the PPE so the athlete can be counseled on the risks and ramifications of injury to the remaining organ. The AAP has issued a guide for athletic participation when there is loss of an organ.[59] This is discussed in more detail in "Determining Clearance," chapter 7 (page 61). In general, absence of a paired organ does not limit the athlete from competing.

◤ VIRAL ILLNESS

28. Have you had infectious mononucleosis (mono) within the last month?

Mononucleosis is a very common illness among 15- to 35-year-olds and is caused by the Epstein-Barr virus.[60] It is transmitted through saliva and mucus, primarily through kissing. Symptoms generally appear 4 to 7 weeks after exposure. Symptoms may be mild or severe and can include severe fatigue, fever, posterior cervical lymphadenopathy, exudative pharyngitis, and left-sided abdominal pain. Atypical activated T lymphocytes (mononuclear cells) appear in the blood. Diagnosis is confirmed with serologic testing or an in-clinic Monospot test.[61] The fatigue associated with mononucleosis may prohibit the athlete from engaging fully in sports for several weeks or months after the onset of symptoms. There is no cure for mononucleosis. Care is supportive, with rest, antipyretics, and analgesics forming the basis of treatment.

Splenomegaly can be present in 50% of patients who have a confirmed diagnosis of mononucleosis and may persist for several weeks after the onset of initial symptoms.[60,61] Recent history of mononucleosis should prompt the physician to evaluate for splenomegaly. The presence of a palpable spleen—one no longer protected by ribs 9 and 10—places the athlete at increased risk for rupture. The athlete, parents or guardians, and coaches should be advised about this risk and adjust activity accordingly.

Even if the spleen is normal size, the architecture remains fragile and susceptible to injury. The AAFP and others recommend that, to minimize the risk of splenic rupture, sports and other physical activities should be avoided for 21 to 28 days weeks after the infection starts.[62,63]

◾ DERMATOLOGIC CONDITIONS

29. Do you have any rashes, pressure sores, or other skin problems?

30. Have you had a herpes skin infection?

Skin conditions can affect participation if the infections are communicable or if the conditions increase the risk of bloodborne pathogens. The NCAA Injury Surveillance System indicates that skin infections are associated with at least 15% of wrestling injuries that result in lost practice time.[64] Skin infections can be easily transmitted in contact or contact-collision sports and are particularly common in wrestling, martial arts, and rugby. This can affect whether athletes will be declared eligible by the rules of their sport at the time of practice or competition.[65,66]

At the time of the PPE, the physician has the opportunity to advise athletes on the signs and symptoms of common skin conditions, whether bacterial, parasitic, viral, or fungal. Common infectious conditions include herpes simplex, tinea, scabies, pubic lice, molluscum contagiosum, furunculosis, carbunculosis, and impetigo.

Isolation of athletes with skin conditions is recommended until appropriate barrier protection and medical intervention has been implemented. Most sports require that competitors completely cover open wounds and infectious skin conditions to prevent exposure to other competitors.[66] This can be very difficult, because sweat can interfere with adherence of tape, bandages, and wraps. Nonetheless, the athlete must be counseled about barrier techniques. The consequences of failure to diagnose and adequately cover skin lesions can be devastating to an athlete, who may be declared ineligible for competition after months of training. Universal precautions are recommended by the CDC for wounds that are open or bleeding.

Early and accurate detection and quarantine from contact until the infection is eradicated with comprehensive treatment are the most effective means of containing an outbreak and minimizing the spread of the disease.[65,66] The NCAA and some high school federations require antibiotics, antivirals, or antifungals for a specified time before participation is permitted.

Prevention strategies include elimination of organisms on mats and equipment, daily change of practice clothing, and immediate showering after practices to reduce the risk of skin infection. Although the primary mode of transmission is through skin-to-skin contact, the ACSM recommends that mats and equipment be cleaned by using a solution of 1 part bleach in 9 parts water.

Herpes gladiatorum is epidemic in wrestlers. The problem can threaten individual wrestlers and even entire teams. Prevention approaches are varied and not standardized.[67] The ACSM and the NFHS are collaborating to develop uniform, evidence-based recommendations.[67,68] On-site precompetition physical examinations screen specifically for this condition, with wrestlers disqualified if they are determined to be infected.

Lesions are vesicular and clustered, generally about the face, neck, and arms. Accompanying symptoms may include sore throat, general malaise, and fever. Season-long prophylactic treatments with antiviral agents for entire teams is increasingly being implemented to prevent widespread infection.[69]

Tinea gladiatorum has been reported to occur in up to 42% of wrestlers.[70] Transmission is via skin-to-skin contact.[71] Preventive measures, including cleansing mats, disinfecting showers, and implementing pharmacologic intervention, are recommended.[71]

Tinea pedis is a fungal infection of the foot. It is extremely common and not a cause for disqualification, unless the participants are barefooted and have open lesions.[72]

Community-acquired methicillin-resistant *Staphylococcus aureus* (MRSA) is being observed in healthy athletes as it is in all outpatient populations. Once entirely focused on relatively minor ailments such as tinea gladiatorum or herpes gladiatorum, sports dermatology is now facing this serious infection, which can have catastrophic consequences.[73] There is no consensus as to why MRSA is being observed in the healthy athletic population, but physicians should be aware of this emerging infection.

MRSA manifests most commonly as a cut or abrasion that has become infected, very painful, extended into adjacent soft tissue, and even developed into an abcess.[73] Fever and chills may be present. Bacteremia may develop. Transmission occurs through skin-to-skin contact and exposure to shared equipment. Transmission control includes hand washing, showering with soap, covering cuts and abrasions, laundering personal items such as towels and supporters, and refraining from sharing razors and towels.

Acne can be difficult to control, even among those athletes being treated, because sweat and constrictive uniforms and equipment may exacerbate the condition. This should not affect eligibility or even performance but may have adverse social and emotional consequences for the athlete.

SECONDARY QUESTIONS

✦ Do you take medication for your skin problem?
✦ Have you ever missed practice or games because of this condition?

◣ NEUROLOGIC CONDITIONS

31. Have you ever had a head injury or concussion?

32. Have you been hit in the head and been confused or lost your memory?

33. Have you ever had a seizure?

34. Do you have headaches with exercise?

35. Have you ever had numbness, tingling, or weakness in your arms or legs after being hit or falling?

36. Have you ever been unable to move your arms or legs after being hit or falling?

A history of a neurologic condition such as seizures; severe and/or recurrent headaches; or trauma resulting in head injuries, concussions, burners or stingers, pinched nerves, or cervical cord neurapraxia (CCN) requires thorough review and will frequently require more evaluation than possible at the PPE screening exam. Such conditions may be an indicator of susceptibility for future catastrophic neurologic injury. Athletes with such history warrant a comprehensive assessment for conditions that may predispose them to undue risk.

Concussions are very common in collision and limited-contact sports. Concussion is, in part, defined as a complex pathophysiologic process affecting the brain, induced by traumatic biomechanical forces[74] or mild traumatic brain injury.[75] The American Academy of Neurology (AAN) defines concussion as trauma-induced alteration in mental status that may or may not involve loss of consciousness.[76]

The incidence of concussion is highest in collision and contact sports such as boxing, ice hockey, football, and soccer. Nine of 10 head injuries in sport are reported as concussions.[77] In football, 20% of high school and 10% of college players sustain concussions annually.[78] Chronic traumatic brain injury may be the consequence of repetitive concussive and subconcussive brain injuries; therefore, query at the PPE is very important in assessing history and risk and formulating preventive strategies.[79]

Signs and symptoms include 1 or more of the following: a brief loss of consciousness, light-headedness, vertigo, cognitive or memory dysfunction, tinnitus, blurred vision, difficulty concentrating, amnesia, headache, nausea, vomiting, photophobia, or a balance disturbance.[80] Confusion and amnesia are hallmarks of concussion.[76] The Standardized Assessment of Concussion (SAC)[81] and Maddocks questions[82] serve to assist in the systematic assessment of an athlete with traumatic brain injury.

Postconcussion syndrome is the persistence of symptoms such as impaired memory or concentration, headache, fatigue, mood swings, sleep disturbances, and dizziness. These symptoms can last a few days or several months.

"Second impact syndrome" (SIS) refers to pancerebral edema associated with traumatic brain injury. The term "second impact syndrome" was coined because the condition was widely thought to be secondary to a primary traumatic brain injury or concussion. This relationship has been questioned, and the entity commonly described as SIS is controversial. The literature suggests that SIS is not necessarily related to a prior head injury but rather may be cerebral edema from a primary brain injury.[83] Concussion guidelines are based, in large part, on the desire to prevent SIS.[83] Further investigation is required to gain a better understanding of traumatic cerebral edema. Future studies may indeed lead us to conclude that SIS is, in fact, the manifestation of a primary injury.

Multiple concussions are a strong cause for concern, because they indicate a susceptibility to permanent brain injury. The PPE should elicit the history of number of concussions or symptoms suggestive of concussion. There are no guidelines for management of an athlete with multiple concussions. Full neurologic evaluation should be done and strong consideration should be made for referral to a specialist familiar with concussions.

The First International Conference on Concussion in Sport, Vienna 2001, recommended that a preparticipation history include specific questions regarding previous symptoms of concussion, not only perceived number of past concussions.[74] This conference recommended that the clinical history also include information about all previous head, face, or neck injuries, as these may have clinical relevance to present or future head injuries. Details regarding the type of protective equipment used at the time of injury should be determined, both for recent and past injuries.[74] An athlete with persistent symptoms associated with concussion at the time of the PPE should not be cleared for participation, and referral to a specialist should be considered.

Amnesia may play a much greater role in determining concussion injury severity than previously recognized.[81] Inquiry into the nature of amnesia and other associated postconcussive symptoms such as headache, fatigue, dizziness, and difficulty with concentration is recommended. Loss of consciousness traditionally has been used as the primary measure of injury severity, but this has limitations in assessing the severity of concussive injury and is increasingly viewed as not being as important as serial neuropsychiatric testing.

Guidelines have been formulated by many organizations for grading concussions based on severity of symptoms.[76,80,84-88] The AAP and AAFP have collaborated to issue recommendations for the management of concussion in athletes age 2 to 20 years.[81] The AAN and the Brain Injury Association of America also have presented information and guidelines.[76,89] Any current guidelines will most certainly undergo revision as knowledge evolves about the neuropathology and neuropsychological sequelae of this injury.

SECONDARY QUESTIONS
- ✦ When did you have your head injury?
- ✦ Did you finish the game or practice?
- ✦ Did you miss any games or practices?
- ✦ Did you see a doctor?
- ✦ Did you have tests like x-rays or a CT scan?
- ✦ Were you ever hospitalized for a head injury?

Seizures are not very common among athletes, in part, because, for many years, patients with this disorder have been discouraged from participating in physical fitness and team sports due to the fear that it will exacerbate their seizure disorder.[90] However, if athletes have good seizure control, they can participate in both collision and contact sports without adversely affecting seizure frequency.[90] Each year, 25,000 to 40,000 children experience their first seizure.[91] A history of new-onset seizure or those occurring after head injury requires thorough review of medical treatment and workup prior to clearance. Antiepileptic drugs have side effects, including rash, hirsutism, weight gain, and nausea. Behavioral and cognitive impairment can also be observed.[91] These side effects and others may affect performance. The World Anti-Doping Agency (WADA) and the NCAA do not ban most antiepileptic drugs, but, as with all medications, athletes should keep up to date with current banned medication lists.

Water sports can present unique challenges for athletes with seizures. Precautions must be taken and risks of drowning discussed. The athlete must never swim or train in the water alone. Athletes should be counseled to inform their physician about any seizure activity so that treatment or workup can be implemented.

Headaches have been reported in up to 51% of 7-year-olds and 82% of 15-year-olds in the general population.[92] In prepuberty, males are more affected than females, but by adolescence the incidence is higher in females.[92] Physicians should consider the most common causes of headaches in the general population as well as sport-specific headaches when evaluating an athlete with headache.

Exercise-associated headaches may be classified by various causes (table 9).[93] They may be an indicator of hypertension, trauma, or another cause.

Migraine headaches frequently develop during adolescence and occur more often in females; 8% to 23% of children age 11 to 15 years report migraine cephalgia.[92] Migraines are not a disqualifier for sports participation but certainly may hamper performance and participation. Migraine cephalgia may occur as a consequence of heightened stress associated with competition, which may be a trigger or may even be associated with previous concussion. Neither WADA nor the NCAA ban ergot derivatives or triptans, commonly used to treat migraine cephalgia, but do ban beta-blockers. Athletes should be questioned about triggers

Table 9	Classification of Exercise-Related Headaches

Exertional—eg, weight lifting or wrestling
Effort—running or aerobic exercise
Posttraumatic—concussion
Cervicogenic—abnormalities of cervical spine anatomy

Adapted with permission from McCrory P: Recognizing exercise-related headache. Phys Sportsmed 1997;25(2):33-43.

so that preventive strategies can be developed.

"Burners" or "stingers" may represent transient brachial plexopathy. Fifty-two percent of college football players experience stingers annually,[94] and, overall, up to 65% have reported at least 1 stinger in their career.[95] Impact to the neck or shoulder causing compression or stretching of the cervical nerve roots (usually C5 or C6) or brachial plexus causes the plexopathy. Athletes experience unilateral upper-extremity burning, stinging, numbness, weakness, or pain. Neurologic signs (weakness) usually disappear rapidly, but symptoms (paresthesias) may linger for several minutes. Only rarely will permanent neurologic sequelae result.[96,97] Motor weakness may even develop hours to days postinjury.[94,95,98]

Isolated stingers are generally considered to be a benign injury, but a history of repeat injury is more concerning. Severe or repeated stingers can lead to long-term muscle weakness with persistent paresthesias.[97,99-101] Query at the PPE should be made to determine the history of isolated or recurrent stingers and whether there are persistent neurologic sequelae.

Up to 87% of football players in 1 study[99] reported recurrent burners. The relative risk of a player experiencing recurrent stingers may be twice that of the risk of a player experiencing an initial stinger.[99] Although there are many contributing factors, cervical spinal stenosis with degenerative disk disease has been postulated to be a prime factor in increasing the risk of recurrent stingers.[101] The history of recurrent stingers does not necessarily preclude participation in collision or contact-collision sports, but athletes with symptoms of recurrent transient brachial plexopathy require investigation for cervical pathology.

Studies to investigate the site and extent of neuropathy, including electromyography and imaging studies, should be considered in these athletes prior to clear-ance for participation in contact-collision sports. Athletes with residual muscle weakness, cervical anomalies, or abnormal electromyographic studies should be excluded from contact sports.[99,102]

Prevention strategies include ensuring properly fitted shoulder pads, considering the use of neck rolls or collars, and reviewing tackling technique.[102,103] Poor tackling technique in football is known to increase the risk for burners and cervical injuries. Rules revised by the NFHS to prohibit "spearing" decreased the incidence of cervical injuries by 60%.[104] The NCAA and others advise athletes with a history of stingers to be instructed about rehabilitation and neck strength training.[104,105]

Cervical cord neurapraxia is a consequence of cervical cord compression, whereby the spinal cord is "pinched," causing increased pressure of and decreased blood flow to the spinal cord.[99,106] CCN manifests as impairment of sensory (burning pain, numbness, or tingling) and/or motor (weakness or paralysis) systems in the extremities. CCN can cause sensory deficits only, sensory deficits with motor weakness, or complete paralysis. Neurologic deficits of CCN can be isolated to bilateral upper extremities, lower extremities or ipsilateral upper and lower extremities.

CCN involving transient quadriplegia is one of the most terrifying on-field situations an athlete or medical staff can encounter in sports. Symptoms usually resolve within 10 to 15 minutes, although some cases resolve gradually over 36 to 48 hours.[97,99,107]

Athletes with normal cervical spine canal diameter and otherwise normal anatomy may sustain neck and cervical spine injury. Transient quadriplegia or spinal cord injury may be found in athletes who have cervical spinal stenosis, congenital fusion, cervical instability, or intervertebral disk protrusion that decreases the anteroposterior cervical spine canal diameter.[99] Although these preexisting anatomic anomalies may predispose an individual to cervical injury, there is much controversy about ascribing risk to individual athletes on the basis of cervical spinal stenosis.

A football player with a history of 1 episode of CCN is more than 900 times more likely to experience a second episode of CCN than an athlete who has never had an episode.[99] The risk of quadriplegic injury after CCN is more than 3,000 times greater than the risk of having a catastrophic neck injury without a previous neck injury. Although return-to-play issues are controversial, most recommend that participation in contact and collision sports be prohibited after the first CCN.[99,108]

If the athlete has had recurrent burners or stingers, transient quadriplegia, or other signs or symptoms of cervical spine pathology, the examiner should determine whether cervical spine radiographs, including flexion and extension views, or further diagnostic studies (eg, MRI) have been performed and what previous recommendations have been given. Further evaluation is indicated for recurrent burners or stingers, unresolved neurologic signs or symptoms, or transient quadriplegia.

SECONDARY QUESTIONS
✦ When did your injury happen?
✦ How did it happen?
✦ Were you taken to a hospital after the injury?
✦ Have you had tests like x-rays or MRI?
✦ Have you missed practices or games because of stingers or neck injury?
✦ Do you have weakness or numbness now?

◾ HEAT ILLNESS

37. When exercising in the heat, do you have severe muscle cramps or become ill?

Heat illness (table 10)[109] adversely affects athletic performance and can be associated with potentially severe morbidity and, occasionally, death from exertional heatstroke. Prior heat illness increases the risk for future heat intolerance or heat illness. The PPE should include specific questions regarding the associated environment, acclimatization status, equipment worn, fluid intake, weight changes during activity, medication and supplement use, and history of cramping or heat illness.[110,111] The preparticipation evaluation is an opportunity for anticipatory guidance, other prevention measures, and treatment strategies.

Risk factors, including young age, poor aerobic fitness, and inadequate acclimatization, may contribute to heat illness (table 11). Other common factors that increase the risk for heat illness include a history of heat illness, dehydration, equipment that inhibits heat loss, excess body fat and large body size, febrile condition, and overexertion.[112] High humidity, even when air temperature is not excessive, may result in high heat stress.[112]

The use of diuretics, caffeine, antihistamines, selec-

Table 10 — Types of Heat-Related Illness

Heat edema
Heat cramps
Heat syncope/exercise-associated collapse
Heat exhaustion
Heatstroke

Table 11 — Possible Factors in Heat-Related Illness

Extrinsic
Sport
Environment
Geography
Clothing and equipment
Certain medications and supplements

Intrinsic
Dehydration
History of heat illness
Inadequate acclimatization
Poor aerobic fitness
Excess body fat
Large body size
Febrile condition
Overexertion
Young age

tive serotonin reuptake inhibitors, second-generation neuroleptics, or methylphenidate (in addition to such drugs as beta-blockers and anticholinergics) increases the risk of heat illness.[109-111] Banned supplements such as ephedra or methamphetamines can also cause dehydration. Athletes should be informed of the increased risk with regard to their medications and supplements.[109]

Children do not adapt to extremes of temperature as effectively as adults when exposed to high climatic heat stress.[112] Children produce less sweat, have fewer sweat glands, and possess a greater body-surface-area-to-body-mass ratio, causing greater heat gain from the environment on a hot day and greater heat loss to the environment on a cold day.[112] They also tend to underestimate body water loss and need encouragement to replace their sweat losses. A commonly used medication for attention deficit disorder, methylphenidate, as noted, can increase the risk of heat-related illness.

Exertional heatstroke and exercise-related col-

lapse in the heat are best prevented by modifying activities in hot, humid conditions to reduce the disparity between body heat production and body heat loss. Normal regulatory mechanisms of heat dissipation can be compromised when uniforms that create a vapor barrier and protective equipment, such as shoulder pads and helmets, are worn.[113] Educating athletes, parents, and coaches about risk factors and preventive strategies is key to decreasing the incidence of heat illness.

SECONDARY QUESTIONS

✦ Did you vomit?
✦ Did you faint?
✦ Did you have cramping?
✦ Did you go to the emergency room?
✦ Did you have an IV?
✦ What medications or supplements do you take?
✦ What do you drink before, during, and after practice or the game?

◣ SICKLE CELL TRAIT OR DISEASE

38. Has a doctor told you that you or someone in your family has sickle cell trait or sickle cell disease?

The focus should be on sickle cell trait, because competitive athletes with sickle cell anemia are unheard of and athletes with sickle cell-thalassemia are rare.

Sickle cell trait occurs in approximately 8% of African Americans and a very small number of Caucasians. In ordinary conditions, sickle cell trait has no life-threatening consequences, carries no additional risk for heat illness in affected athletes, and does not increase the risk of exertional heat illness.[114] However, recent case reports of sudden death in athletes with sickle cell trait during strenuous activity in the heat or at higher altitudes have rightly caused concern.[59] Black athletes should be questioned about whether they have sickle cell trait and counseled on recommendations for sports in the face of the risk of sudden death from sickling during strenuous activity, especially in the heat or at altitude.

The US Armed Forces reported more than a 20-fold increase in risk of death among recruits with sickle cell trait engaged in strenuous activity compared with controls without sickle cell trait.[115,116]

While extreme conditions increase the risk of sickling, it can happen any time an athlete does a "heroic" workout like racing the clock to make the team. Death occurs not from heatstroke but from the complications of sickling, including fulminant ischemic rhabdomyolysis, profound metabolic acidosis, acute renal failure, and multiple-organ system failure.[114]

Athletes with sickle cell trait are advised to avoid strenuous activity that leads to muscle pain, such as early-season football and basketball sprints beyond 500 m (cumulative sum).[59,117] The combined forces of profound hypoxemia, acidosis, hyperthermia, and red blood cell (RBC) dehydration in the microcirculation of the working muscles causes the red cell proteins to sickle, and 1 study[118] did observe an increase in sickled RBCs in venous blood after aerobic exercise.

It is recommended that athletes with sickle cell trait acclimatize gradually and engage in year-round training to maintain physical conditioning. Athletes should be instructed on the importance of preventing dehydration, including maintaining adequate fluid intake, avoiding diuretics, and avoiding all-out sprints or timed miles early in training.[119]

◣ EYES AND VISION

39. Have you had any problems with your eyes or vision?

40. Do you wear glasses or contact lenses?

41. Do you wear protective eyewear, such as goggles or a face shield?

Visual acuity must be assessed and documented at the time of the PPE. The AAP recommends vision screening at all well-child visits.[120] Vision can slowly deteriorate over time without the athlete being aware of the changes. Poor vision can lead to poor performance and injuries.

Eye protection is key to preventing eye injuries. In 2000, there were 42,000 eye injuries related to sports and recreation, and more than 50% occurred in those under 15 years old.[121] The AAP and the American Academy of Ophthalmology (AAO) strongly recommend protective eyewear for all participants in sports in which there is risk of eye injury.[122] The NFHS mandates the use of protective eyewear for high school girls' lacrosse, and US Lacrosse will mandate use beginning in 2005.[123] USA Hockey requires face shields for eye protection.[124] The AAO reports that significant eye injury can be reduced at least 90% when properly fitted, appropriate eye protectors are used.[125-127]

The sports with the highest risk of eye injury are baseball and basketball. Risk for injury in a particular sport is categorized into high, moderate, low, and eye safe (see table 24 on page 70).[122] Sports with balls or those with a likely risk of participants' being hit are considered to be high risk (eg, softball, martial arts). Track and gymnastics are two sports considered "eye safe."

Lenses made of polycarbonate or CR-39 are recommended for protection. Standard eyeglasses with plastic or glass lenses commonly worn to correct vision are not considered adequate protection against eye injury in sports. The AAP recommends that even in low–eye-risk sports, athletes use at least approved street-wear frames that meets American National Standards Institute (ANSI) standard Z87.1 with polycarbonate or CR-39 lenses. A strap must secure the frame to the head and must be fitted by an experienced ophthalmologist, optometrist, or optician. For high–eye-risk sports, the AAP recommends full sports goggles made of polycarbonate.[120] A list of specific sports and recommendations for eyewear can be obtained from the AAP Committee on Sports Medicine and Fitness (see table 25 on page 71). Athletes must be cautioned that contact lenses do not confer any protection from injury and must not be considered eye protectors.

Athletes with best-corrected visual acuity in 1 eye worse than 20/40 (eg, 20/100) are considered "functionally one-eyed." The AAO and the AAP recommend mandatory protective eyewear for all functionally one-eyed athletes regardless of sport. Athletes who have had an eye injury or surgery may have a globe that is weakened and therefore more susceptible to injury. The AAO states that such athletes and those who are functionally 1-eyed must not participate in boxing, wrestling, or full-contact martial arts.

SECONDARY QUESTIONS

✦ When was your last eye examination?

✦ Why don't you wear eye protection? (if applicable)

✦ Have you had eye surgery (eg, PRK, LASIK)?

◥ NUTRITIONAL CONCERNS

42. Are you happy with your weight?

43. Are you trying to gain or lose weight?

44. Has anyone recommended you change your weight or eating habits?

45. Do you limit or carefully control what you eat?

Nutrition is very important in optimizing performance. It is well documented that some athletes, especially those in sports in which "making weight" is important and those with subjective judging, do not have adequate caloric intake. The underweight and undernourished athlete is a concern. Conversely, the overweight and poorly nourished athlete should also be a concern, especially in light of overwhelming epidemiologic evidence of increasing childhood and adult obesity and the comorbidities associated with this disease. The PPE is an opportune time to engage in a discussion about nutrition and weight.[128]

Disordered eating in the adolescent and athletic population is increasing.[7] This includes a spectrum of unhealthy nutritional behaviors from inadvertent (ie, poor nutritional habits) or calculated calorie deprivation, self-induced vomiting, laxative use, diuretic use, anorexia nervosa, and bulimia nervosa to overeating. Disordered eating with calorie deprivation is most prevalent in athletes participating in sports with weight classes (eg, wrestling, rowing [crew], and judo), sports in which judging may be influenced by appearance (eg, gymnastics, figure skating, diving, dancing, and cheerleading) and sports emphasizing leanness for optimal performance (eg, track and field, distance running).[128,129]

Eating disorders are most common among female athletes (10:1).[130] At any given time, 10% or more of college-aged women report symptoms of eating disorders. Although these symptoms may not satisfy full diagnostic criteria, they do often cause distress.[130] Interventions with these individuals may be helpful and may prevent the development of more serious disorders.[130]

Frequently, athletes falsify information about nutrition to mask weight-loss techniques. Fears of restricted athletic participation, loss of self-control, and uncovering of underlying personal stressors may make athletes leery of providing accurate information, so a useful history may be difficult to obtain.

BMI is a tool for indicating weight status[131] and correlates with body fat. The relation between fatness and BMI differs with age and gender.[132] In children and teens, BMI is referred to as, "BMI-for-age" and is gender and age specific. BMI-for-age is plotted on gender-specific growth charts for children and teens age 2 to 20 years.[132] Straight-calculated BMI is used to determine the weight status for adults over 20 years of age, without regard to gender or age.

BMI-for-age at less than the 5th percentile is considered underweight for children and teens, and BMI less than 18.5 is classified as underweight for adults older than 20 years by the CDC and the World Health Organization.[132] Athletes below this value must be counseled about proper weight and nutrition and asked about emotions related to food. All underweight athletes should be referred to a nutritionist, and strong consideration should be made for referral to a psychologist or psychiatrist for a workup and specific diagnosis. These are best made by clinicians on the basis of specific criteria from *The Diagnostic and Statistical Manual of Mental Disorders,* Fourth Edition, Text Revision (DSM-IV-TR).[130]

SECONDARY QUESTIONS

✦ How much would you like to weigh?

✦ In the last year, what was your highest weight? Lowest weight?

✦ Have you ever tried diet pills, sitting in a sauna, diuretics, laxatives, vomiting, or similar techniques to lose weight?

✦ What exercises do you do in addition to training for your sport?*

*This final secondary question may elicit a response indicating the athlete might be overtraining, which may lead to overuse injuries and also excessive weight loss and menstrual disorders. The female athlete triad can lead to catastrophic medical and emotional consequences and is frequently seen in underweight athletes, such as runners, who do not take in adequate calories to support their training regimen.

Overweight in children and adolescents is an increasing concern (see, "Defining Overweight Children," at right). According to the AAP, 15.3% of 6- to 11-year-olds and 15.5% of 12- to 19-year-olds are at or above the 95th percentile for BMI.[32,132] This is a significant risk factor for comorbities, including type 2 diabetes,

hypertension, dyslipidemia, and other metabolic disorders. Sports and increased physical activity, along with prudent dietary intake, is the "cure" for this epidemic, so these steps should be emphasized in this at-risk group. It should be noted that lean individuals with a high body muscle mass may not necessarily be overweight or obese. Individual consideration of body habitus should be made when using the BMI as one tool of an overall health risk assessment to prohibit the inaccurate labeling of an athlete based on weight classification.

The PPE is a good time for physicians to assess the need for further workup, such as laboratory testing for dyslipidemia or for diabetes. If a young athlete has a BMI greater than the 85th percentile for age and gender, a follow-up visit to screen for hypertension, dyslipidemia, and other comorbidities is indicated.[133]

The social stigma and emotional pain associated with being overweight cannot be overstated and may have lifelong consequences.[134] The PPE is an opportunity for physicians to encourage young overweight athletes to continue their athletic pursuits and emphasize the importance of lifelong physical activity. A review of sound nutritional habits with suggestions for modifications that promote a healthy lifestyle is strongly recommended.[135,136]

DEFINING OVERWEIGHT CHILDREN

The CDC defines overweight in children differently than for adults. For children over age 10, overweight is defined as:

✦ BMI greater than the 95th percentile for age and gender;

✦ Weight-for-height ratio 95th percentile; and

✦ Weight greater than 20% of ideal weight for height.

Those at risk for being overweight are those with:

✦ BMI from the 85th to 95th percentile for age and gender; and

✦ Weight-for-height ratio between the 85th and 95th percentiles.

BMI charts for children can be obtained from the CDC at www.cdc.gov/growthcharts.

GENERAL CONCERNS

46. Do you have any concerns that you would like to discuss with a doctor?

The final history question for both sexes is an open invitation to discuss any matter privately and confidentially with the physician. The follow-up questions beginning on page 36 are based on questions from the YRBSS and may give the physician greater insight into the athlete's mental health and also into any high-risk behaviors.

MENSTRUAL HISTORY

47. Have you ever had a menstrual period?
48. How old were you when you had your first menstrual period?
49. How many periods have you had in the last 12 months?

Menstrual history is important for female athletes, because disordered menses may be a sign of disordered eating, pregnancy, or other gynecologic or metabolic condition. A detailed menstrual history is important if answers to any of the first primary questions indicate a possible menstrual problem.

Amenorrhea, both primary and secondary, should be detected by history. Primary amenorrhea is defined as the absence of menarche at age 16. Secondary amenorrhea refers to missing at least 3 consecutive menstrual periods in a previously menstruating female; the most common cause is pregnancy.

Athletes who are underweight (BMI < 18.5) should be assessed for nutritional status. Low body fat can be a factor in the development of amenorrhea and oligomenorrhea (ie, periods that occur at intervals greater than every 35 days). Runners and athletes in sports where low weight is thought to be advantageous (eg, gymnasts, figure skaters) are particularly susceptible to menstrual irregularities.

Athletes with amenorrhea or oligomenorrhea should be referred to their primary care physician or to a gynecologist for further evaluation. A search for other causes of menstrual disturbance, such as pregnancy, should be undertaken before attributing amenorrhea to the female athlete triad or to excessive exercise. Problems that may accompany exercise-associated amenorrhea include poor nutrition, inadequate bone mineralization, and stress fractures.

Hypermenorrhea or polymenorrhea may lead to blood loss and iron deficiency, resulting in anemia, fa-

tigue, and poor athletic performance. Hypermenorrhea is defined as excessively prolonged or profuse menses. Polymenorrhea is having menstrual cycles of greater-than-usual frequency. If these conditions are present, coordination of care for further workup to determine the underlying cause and for investigation of possible anemia is strongly recommended. Physical signs include pale conjunctiva, rapid pulse, and high-output flow murmur.

The physician should inquire about recent Pap tests in females who are over age 18 or who are sexually active, and advise the athlete to see her personal physician for health maintenance, Pap testing, and instruction in breast self-examination.

SECONDARY QUESTIONS
✦ How much time do you usually have from the start of 1 period to the start of another?
✦ What was the longest time between periods in the last year?

IMMUNIZATIONS

Most school districts require standard immunizations for entrance—for example, tetanus, measles, mumps, rubella, diphtheria, pertussis, chickenpox, polio, Haemophilus influenzae, and hepatitis B.[72] For a list of immunizations required for school entry by state, visit www.immunizationinfo.org/vaccineInfo/index.cfm#state.

Whether or not an athlete is up to date regarding immunizations does not affect athletic eligibility. However, the PPE is an opportunity to inquire about the status of elective, but recommended, immunizations such hepatitis B and influenza A (table 12).[69] Athletes should be informed of the risk of missed practices and games as a result of contracting influenza A, especially for the winter sports in which the proximity of players, coaches, and other team personnel during "flu season" from November to February makes contracting influenza much easier, with potentially devastating effects for the team. Other diseases of concern for athletes for which there are vaccines include hepatitis A and meningococcal meningitis.[72,137] Athletes traveling internationally may have specific vaccination needs, and athletes starting college in a dormitory setting should receive menigococcal vaccine (table 13).[137]

Athletes with chronic illnesses such as diabetes, asth-

Table 12 — Recommended Immunizations for Adolescent and Adult Athletes

Vaccine	Initial Dosage/Booster	Contraindications
Strongly Recommended		
Tetanus /diphtheria	3 primary doses, followed by booster in 3-4 yr and boosters every 10 yr thereafter	Anaphylaxis to vaccine; significant illness in progress
Measles, mumps, rubella	2 doses: first after age 12 mo, second at least 30 days later	Anaphylaxis or severe allergy to vaccine; significant illness in progress; immunocompromised state
Hepatitis B	3 doses: initial, 1 mo later, and 6 mo later	Hypersensitivity to yeast or other vaccine component
Influenza	Single annual trivalent dose	Allergy to eggs or other vaccine components
Poliomyelitis	2 doses at 1-2 mo interval; 1 more dose 6-12 mo later	Hypersensitivity to neomycin, streptomycin sulfate, or polymyxin B sulfate; acute febrile illness
To Be Considered		
Hepatitis A	First dose at least 2 wk before exposure; booster 6-12 mo later	Severe reaction to vaccine or components
Pneumococcal (23-valent)	Single dose	Avoid giving for 2 wk after immunosuppressive therapy; active infection
Meningococcal	Single dose	Hypersensitivity to components; acute illness
Varicella	2 doses, 4-8 wk apart	Hypersensitivity to gelatin or neomycin; bone marrow or lymphatic malignancy

*For athletes traveling to foreign competitions, consider necessary vaccines, such as yellow fever, typhoid fever, cholera, Japanese encephalitis, and rabies.

For up-to-date immunization guidelines, see www.cdc.gov/nip/recs/child-schedule.htm or www.cdc.gov/nip/recs/teen-schedule.htm#chart.

Reprinted with permission from: Howe WB Preventing infectious disease in sports. Phys Sportsmed 2003;31(2):23-29.

ma, or cystic fibrosis may benefit from pneumococcus vaccine in addition to the influenza immunization.

◣ QUESTIONS FOR THE FOLLOW-UP INTERVIEW

1. Do you feel stressed out or under a lot of pressure?

2. Do you ever feel so sad or hopeless that you stop doing some of your usual activities for more than a few days?

3. Do you feel safe?

4. Have you ever tried cigarette smoking, even 1 or 2 puffs? Do you currently smoke?

5. During the past 30 days, did you use chewing tobacco, snuff, or dip?

6. During the past 30 days, have you had at least 1 drink of alcohol?

7. Have you ever taken steroid pills or shots without a doctor's prescription?

Adverse Reactions	Comments
Local reactions, fever	Current problems with vaccine supply have temporarily modified recommendations
Fever, rash, transient thrombocytopenia (rare)	Required by most schools and colleges
Local reactions, fever	Important for healthcare personnel, including athletic trainers; universal immunization is a goal
Local reactions	Important for adult team sports during flu season; minimal risk of Guillain-Barré syndrome since swine flu vaccine
Local reaction, fever	Only inactivated virus used in USA; important for travel to polio-infected areas*
Local reactions, headache, malaise	Inject into deltoid; consider for travel to endemic areas*
Local reactions, fever	Important for people who are older, immunocompromised, or splenectomized
Mild, localized erythema	Splenectomized patients; consider for travel to endemic areas in December-June*; recommended for college students living in dorms
Local reactions, fever, rash	Patients older than 12 yr who have not had childhood disease

8. Have you ever taken any supplements to help you gain or lose weight or improve your performance?

9. Questions from the Youth Risk Behavior Survey on guns, seatbelts, unprotected sex, domestic violence, drugs, etc.

These follow-up questions are based on those of the YRBSS, which was developed by the CDC in 1990 to monitor priority health risk behaviors that contribute markedly to the leading causes of death, disability, and social problems among youth and adults in the United States. Data are compiled from surveys of representative samples of 9th through 12th grade students every 2 years.[7,138] They are also based on Healthy People 2010 findings and goals.[139]

Athletes may have medical or social concerns that they do not feel comfortable documenting on the official form, but about which they would like advice. The questions are designed to invite conversation between the physician and athlete about social concerns that may affect the athlete's overall heath and well-being. They are not listed on the history form and may be best brought up during the physical examination, which is why they are listed on that form (page 94). The intent is to give the athlete an opportunity to ask questions and address concerns in a nonthreatening, confidential environment.

Many schools require student-athletes to sign a contract or agreement attesting that they will not drink alcohol or use tobacco, illicit drugs, or other banned substances. "Zero tolerance" places the offending athlete at risk of immediate dismissal from the athletic team. This risk of dismissal can certainly have the effect of stifling athletes who have a problem or at-risk behavior from being truthful and seeking counseling.

Therefore, we have also included, as an attachment, a "Teen Screen," which is designed as a tool to invite conversation between the physician and young athlete (see page 98). The "Teen Screen" is not intended to be included in the record of the PPE but rather serve as a template upon which conversation can be based. The athlete should be assured that any conversation is entirely confidential and coaches will not have access to this information. Athletes should be assured that the physician is an advocate for them and only wishes to listen and provide information so they can make healthy choices.

1. Do you feel stressed out or under a lot of pressure?

2. Do you ever feel so sad or hopeless that you stop doing some of your usual activities for more than a few days?

3. Do you feel safe?

Mental health is an important aspect to the overall health assessment of the athlete. Suicide is the third-leading cause of death among youth and young adults age 15 to 24.[140] Students can feel under extreme pressure to perform well in athletics even as they cope with other stresses of adolescence. These primary questions may elicit responses suggestive of depression and provide insight into the psychological well-being of the athlete,

Table 13 — Recommended Vaccinations for International Travelers

Vaccine	Dosage	Length of Immunity
Hepatitis A	Havrix: 1 mL IM at 0 and 6 mo Vaqta: 1 mL IM at 0 and 6 mo	≥10 yr ≥10 yr
Hepatitis B	Energix B: 1 mL IM at 0, 1, and 6 mo* Recombivax: 1 mL IM at 0, 1, and 6 mo*	Need for booster not established Need for booster not established
Influenza	0.5 mL IM single dose given before flu season	1 yr
Japanese B encephalitis	1 mL SC at 0, 7 days later, and 30 days after initial dose	3 yr
Measles, mumps, rubella	0.5 mL SC at 0 and 1 mo	No booster recommended
Meningococcal meningitis	0.5 mL SC single dose	Booster recommended every 3-5 yr, if at risk
Pneumococcal	0.5 mL IM or SC single dose	A booster dose can be given after 5 yr
Poliomyelitis IPV	0.5 mL SC single dose	If primary series has been completed in childhood, a one-time booster received during adulthood provides immunity for life
Rabies	Imovax HDCV: 1 mL at initial, 7 days later, and 21 days after initial dose	If at risk, booster recommended or antibody testing every 2 yr
Tetanus and diphtheria toxoid	0.5 mL IM single dose	If primary series has been completed, booster recommended every 5-10 yr
Typhoid	Ty21a: 1 capsule orally every other day for 4 doses TyphimVi: 0.5 mL IM	Booster every 5 yr Booster every 2 yr
Varicella	Varivax: 0.5 mL SC at 0 and 4-8 wk later	Booster not recommended
Yellow fever	0.5 mL SC single dose †	Booster every 10 yr if needed for travel

*Accelerated schedule at 0, 1, and 2 mo, but requires a booster at 12 mo for full immunity.
†Contraindicated if history of anaphylaxis to egg.
IM = intramuscular injection; SC = subcutaneous injection; IPV = inactivated polio virus; HDCV = human diploid cell vaccine

For up-to-date travel immunization guidelines by country, see http://www.cdc.gov/travel/vaccinat.htm.

Reprinted with permission from: Jiménez CE: Preparing active patients for international travel. Phys Sportsmed 2003;31(10): 27-35.

which may lead to referral for further counseling.

Athletes who are taking medication for depression may find their stamina affected. They may feel stigmatized by their depression. Discussion in a private, non-threatening environment is best.

The "Do you feel safe?" question is suggested to screen for violence, whether or not the provider suspects that abuse has occurred. The adolescent athlete should be interviewed without parents or guardians present to promote candor.

4. Have you ever tried cigarette smoking, even 1 or 2 puffs? Do you currently smoke?

Tobacco use is considered the chief preventable cause of death in the United States, with approximately one fifth of all deaths attributable to its use. Cigarette smoking is responsible for heart disease; cancers of the lung, larynx, mouth, esophagus, and bladder; stroke; and chronic obstructive pulmonary disease. In addition, cigarette smokers are more likely to drink alcohol and use marijuana and cocaine as compared with nonsmokers. In 2003, cigarette use among high school students was 21.9%.[141]

5. During the past 30 days, did you use chewing tobacco, snuff, or dip?

This question measures smokeless tobacco use. Smokeless tobacco use primarily begins in early adolescence. Approximately 75% of oral cavity and pharyngeal cancers are attributed to the use of smoked and smokeless tobacco. In 2001, 14.8% of male high school students were current smokeless tobacco users.[139]

Many athletes use smokeless tobacco under the mistaken belief that it will improve athletic performance. There is no evidence to support this. Smokeless tobacco does increase heart rate but does not affect reaction time, movement time, or total response time.[142] Tobacco use may be associated with a decrease in maximum voluntary force and maximum rate of force generation.[142] In fact, there is no evidence to support the claim by athletes that neuromuscular performance is enhanced by the use of smokeless tobacco.

The NCAA bans the use of tobacco products by student-athletes and game personnel during practice and competition because of their harmful health effects. The NFHS Coaches Code of Ethics states that coaches shall avoid the use of alcohol and tobacco products when in contact with players.[143]

6. During the past 30 days, have you had at least 1 drink of alcohol?

The CDC reports that 44.9% of youth age 15 to 19 drank alcohol on at least 1 occasion during the past 30 days.[139] Alcohol affects coordination, impairs judgment, and usually does not enhance athletic performance. Motor vehicle crashes are the leading cause of death among youth 15 to 19 years old in the United States, and approximately 30% of all motor vehicle crashes that result in injury involve alcohol.[7] Athletes should be advised against driving while intoxicated or riding in a car with an intoxicated driver. In 2003, 12.1% of high school students nationwide reported having driven a vehicle 1 or more times after drinking alcohol in the past 30 days, and 30.2% of high school students report-

ed riding on 1 or more occasions in the past 30 days in a car with a driver who had been drinking alcohol.[139]

Heavy drinking among youth also has been linked to more sexual partners, elevated marijuana use, and poorer academic performance.[139] In 2003, 44.9% of 15- to 19-year-olds had 1 or more drinks of alcohol in the past 30 days, and 28.3% had 5 or more drinks of alcohol on 1 or more occasions during the past 30 days.[139]

NCAA guidelines stipulate that athletic departments conduct a drug and alcohol education program once a semester to inform athletes of NCAA and institutional drug and alcohol policies.[144] The WADA and the United States Anti-Doping Agency (USADA) prohibit using alcohol during competition in several sports, including archery, soccer, gymnastics, and wrestling. It is considered ergogenic in sports such as archery in which slowed responses may be beneficial.[145,146] The ACSM has issued a position stand about alcohol use among athletes.[147]

7. Have you ever taken steroid pills or shots without a doctor's prescription?

Adolescents often receive mixed signals about the benefits and risks of anabolic steroids. Physicians must be familiar with incentives and disincentives for use.

Anabolic steroids are banned by every major governing body, including the International Olympic Committee, US Olympic Committee,[148] and NCAA.[149] USA Track and Field has issued a "death penalty," or lifelong ban, from the sport for first-time steroid offenses. The National Football League (NFL) has strict policies against anabolic steroid use and performs random year-round testing.

On the other hand, Major League Baseball has a very lax policy. This sends mixed signals to young athletes, who frequently emulate professionals. Reports have shown that 6% to 11% of high school athletes and 2.2% of junior high athletes are using anabolic steroids, synthetic derivatives of testosterone.[150]

Manifestations of use. A sudden increase in weight or the development of hypertension may be signs of anabolic steroid use.[151] Physical characteristics of steroid use can include gynecomastia, testicular atrophy, hirsutism, alopecia, and excessive acne. Aggressive behavior, depression, anxiety, frequent mood swings, irritability, and libido changes may also be noted.[151] Anabolic steroids can cause hypercoagulability, leading to increased incidence of life-threatening complications from pulmonary embolus, cerebrovascular accidents, sudden cardiac death, coronary thrombus, myocardial infarction, and, ultimately, congestive heart failure and/or cardiomyopathy.[151,152] Anabolic steroids have also been associated with premature closure of the growth plates of long bones. Tumors involving the brain, liver, and kidneys also have been linked to anabolic steroid use.[151]

Targeted counseling. Although it is naïve to expect that the athlete will admit to steroid use, the PPE is an opportunity to inquire and counsel the athlete about peer pressure, health risks, and threat to eligibility. It is impractical to take a history to cover every abused substance or steroid "du jour," but awareness of local trends will guide counseling. Athletes should be reassured that conversations are confidential and that the physician is their advocate. These inquiries may be included as part of the "Teen Screen" (page 98).

8. Have you ever taken any supplements to help you gain or lose weight or improve your performance?

Nutritional or dietary supplements are a concern for two primary reasons: safety and eligibility. The US Food and Drug Administration (FDA) does not strictly regulate the supplement industry; therefore, purity and safety of nutritional supplements cannot be guaranteed (table 14).[153] Athletes should be informed that steroids and other banned substances have been found to contaminate some over-the-counter supplements, and coaches and parents or guardians need to understand this as well. Athletes use these substances at their own risk. Some previously commonly used substances such as ephedrine have been banned by the FDA, but only after many reports of adverse effects and some deaths.

Ergogenic aids are drugs, techniques, substances, or devices used to enhance performance. Ergogenic substances, used for centuries by athletes trying to gain an edge on the competition, have become very sophisticated, and their use is not limited to elite athletes.

Physicians have a duty to inquire about the use of

Table 14	World Anti-Doping Agency Prohibited Classes of Substances

Stimulants
Narcotics
Cannabinoids
Anabolic agents
Peptide hormones
Beta-2 agonists
Agents with antiestrogenic activity (for males)
Masking agents
Glucocorticosteroids

any medications or supplements and advise athletes to be aware of the drug-testing policies of their sport. Athletes must be aware of the names and dosages of drugs and supplements they are taking and the policies applicable to them from their NGB. The NCAA and other NGBs place the responsibility of knowing what athletes are taking entirely on the athlete.

Supplements may contain substances not listed on the package label that may be banned by the sport's NGB. Use of such banned substances, either intentionally or unintentionally, may jeopardize the athlete's eligibility. The NCAA,[149] USADA,[154] and WADA[155] all have documents listing banned substances to assist athletes and physicians.

9. Questions from the Youth Risk Behavior Survey on guns, seatbelts, unprotected sex, domestic violence, drugs, etc.

The CDC's YRBSS (www.cdc.gov/yrbss) provides national, state, and local data on the prevalence of 6 categories of priority health risk behaviors. The YRBSS provides the CDC, states, and others with vital information to more effectively target and evaluate programs. State and local education agencies use data from the YRBSS to inform policymakers about the need for interventions in their jurisdictions to help young people avoid risk behaviors. The queries are from the Youth Risk Behavior Survey, a component of the YRBSS.

REFERENCES
1. Risser WL, Hoffman HM, Bellah GG Jr: Frequency of preparticipation sports examinations in secondary school athletes: are the University Interscholastic League guidelines appropriate? Tex Med 1985;81(7):35-39
2. Goldberg B, Saraniti A, Witman P, et al: Pre-participation sports assessment an objective evaluation. Pediatrics

1980;66(5):736-745
3. Maron BJ, Thompson PD, Puffer JC, et al: Cardiovascular preparticipation screening of competitive athletes: a statement for health professionals from the Sudden Death Committee (clinical cardiology) and Congenital Cardiac Defects Committee (cardiovascular disease in the young), American Heart Association. Circulation 1996;94(4):850-856

4. Metzl JD: Expectations of pediatric sport participation among pediatricians, patients, and parents. Pediatr Clin North Am June 2002;49(3):497-504

5. Maron BJ, Poliac LC, Roberts WO: Risk for sudden cardiac death associated with marathon running. J Am Coll Cardiol 1996;28(2):428-431

6. American Academy of Pediatrics Ad Hoc Task Force on Definition of the Medical Home: the medical home. Pediatrics 1992;90(5):774

7. Grunbaum JA, Kann L, Kinchen S, et al: Youth risk behavior surveillance—United States, 2001. MMWR Surveill Summ 2002;51(4):1-62

8. Kurowski K, Chandran S: The preparticipation athletic evaluation. Am Fam Physician 2000;61(9):2683-2690, 2696-2698

9. Metzl JD: Preparticipation examination of the adolescent athlete: part 1. Pediatr Rev June 2001;22(6):199-204

10. Increased risk of achilles tendon rupture with quinolone antibacterial use, especially in elderly patients taking oral corticosteroids. Infect Dis Clin Pract 2004;12(2):146-147

11. Kowatari K, Nakashima K, Ono A, et al: Levofloxacin-induced bilateral Achilles tendon rupture: a case report and review of the literature. J Orthop Sci 2004;9(2):186-190

12. Hosey RG, Carek PJ, Goo A: Exercise-induced anaphylaxis and urticaria. Am Fam Physician 2001;64(8):1367-1372

13. 26th Bethesda Conference: Recommendations for determining eligibility for competition in athletes with cardiovascular abnormalities. J Am Coll Cardiol 1996;24(4): 867-899 (Task Forces 1-6)

14. Maron BJ, Shirani J, Poliac LC, et al: Sudden death in young competitive athletes: clinical, demographic, and pathological profiles. JAMA 1996;276(3):199-204

15. Van Camp SP, Bloor CM, Mueller FO, et al: Nontraumatic sports deaths in high school and college athletes. Med Sci Sports Exerc 1995;27(5):641-647

16. Basilico FC: Cardiovascular disease in athletes. Am J Sports Med 1999;27(1):108-121

17. Liberthson RR: Sudden death from cardiac causes in children and young adults. N Engl J Med 1996;334(16):1039-1044

18. Luckstead EF Sr: Cardiac risk factors and participation guidelines for youth sports. Pediatr Clin North Am 2002; 49(4):681-707

19. Maron BJ: Risk profiles and cardiovascular preparticipation screening of competitive athletes. Cardiol Clin 1997;15:(3) 473-483

20. Thompson PD, Funk EJ, Carleton RA, et al: Incidence of death during jogging in Rhode Island from 1975 through 1980. JAMA 1982;247(18):2535-2538

21. Mounsey JP, Ferguson JD: The assessment and management of arrhythmias and syncope in the athlete. Clin Sports Med 2003;22(1):67-79

22. Driscoll DJ, Edwards WD: Sudden unexpected death in children and adolescents. J Am Coll Cardiol 1985;5 (6 suppl):118B-121B

23. Pyeritz RE: The Marfan syndrome. Annu Rev Med 2000; 51:481-510

24. Patel DR, Greydanus DE: The adolescent athlete: assessment for sports participation, in Hofmann AD, Greydanus DE (ed): Adolescent Medicine, ed 3. Stamford, CT, Appleton & Lange, 1997, p 608

25. Wiens L, Sabath R, Ewing L, et al: Chest pain in otherwise healthy children and adolescents is frequently caused by exercise-induced asthma. Pediatrics 1992;90(3):350-353

26. Selbst SM: Consultation with the specialist: Chest pain in children. Pediatr Rev 1997;18(5):169-173

27. Kaplan NM, Deveraux RB, Miller HS Jr: 26th Bethesda Conference: recommendations for determining eligibility for competition in athletes with cardiovascular abnormalities, Task Force 4: systemic hypertension. J Am Coll Cardiol. 1994;24(4):885-888

28. DiFiori JP, Haney S: Preparticipation evaluation of collegiate athletes. Med Sci Sports Exerc 2004;36(5):S102, abstracted

29. Vogt BA: Hypertension in children and adolescents: definition, pathophysiology, risk factors and long-term sequelae. Current Therap Res 2001;62:283-297

30. Working Group on Hypertension Control in Children and Adolescents: Update on the 1987 Task Force Report on High Blood Pressure in Children and Adolescents: a working group report from the National High Blood Pressure Education Program. Pediatrics 1996;98(4 pt 1):649-658

31. American Academy of Pediatrics Committee on Sports Medicine and Fitness: Athletic Participation by children and adolescents who have systemic hypertension. Pediatrics 1997;99(4):637-638

32. Krebs NF, Jacobson MS, American Academy of Pediatrics Committee on Nutrition: Prevention of pediatric overweight and obesity. Pediatrics 2003;112(2):424-430

33. American Diabetes Association: Type 2 diabetes in children and adolescents. Diabetes Care 2000;23(3):381-389

34. Danford DA, McNamara DG: Innocent murmurs and heart sounds, in Garson A Jr, Bricker JT, McNamara DG (eds): The Science and Practice of Pediatric Cardiology, ed 2. Baltimore, Williams & Wilkins, 1998

35. Harris, JP: Consultation with the specialist: Evaluation of heart murmurs. Pediatr Rev 1994;15(12):490-493

36. Rosenthal A: How to distinguish between innocent and pathologic murmurs in childhood. Pediatr Clin North Am 1984;31(6):1229-1240

37. Luckstead EF: Cardiovascular evaluation of the young athlete. Adolesc Med 1998;9(3):441-455

38. Friedman RA. Myocarditis, in Garson A, Bricker JT, (eds): The Science and Practice of Pediatric Cardiology. Philadelphia: Lippincott, Williams and Wilkins, 2000

39. Glover DW, Maron BJ: Profile of preparticipation cardiovascular screening for high school athletes. JAMA 1998;279(22):1817-1819

40. Lyznicki JM, Nielsen NH, Schneider JF: Cardiovascular screening of student athletes. Am Fam Physician 2000;62(4):765-774; erratum 2001;63(12):2332

41. Hosey RG, Armsey TD: Sudden cardiac death. Clin Sports Med 2003;22(1):51-66

42. Brukner P, Bradshaw C, Bennell K: Managing common stress fractures: let risk level guide treatment. Phys Sportsmed 1998;26(8):39-47

43. Marx RG, Saint-Phard D, Callahan LR, et al: Stress fracture sites related to underlying bone health in athletic females. Clin J Sport Med 2001;11(2):73-76

44. Harmon KG: Lower extremity stress fractures. Clin J Sport Med 2003;13(6):358-364

45. Chang FM: The disabled athlete, in Stanitiski CL: Pediatric and Adolescent Sports Medicine, vol 3 of Orthopaedic Sports Medicine: Principles and Practice. Philadelphia, WB Saunders, 1994, pp 48-75

46. Braganza SF: Atlantoaxial dislocation. Pediatr Rev 2003;24(3):106-107

47. American Academy of Pediatrics Committee on Sports Medicine and Fitness: Atlantoaxial instability in Down Syndrome: subject review. Pediatrics 1995;96(1 pt 1):151-154

48. Svensson O, Aaro S: Cervical instability in skeletal dysplasia: Report of 6 surgically fused cases. Acta Orthop Scand 1988;59(1):66-70

49. Special Olympics Web site: http://www.specialolympics.org. Accessed August 6, 2004

50. Martin TJ, American Academy of Pediatrics Committee on Sports Medicine and Fitness: Technical report: knee brace use in the young athlete. Pediatrics 2001;108(2):503-507

51. American Academy of Orthopedic Surgeons: Position statement: the use of knee braces. Available at

http://www.aaos.org/wordhtml/papers/position/1124.htm. Accessed August 9, 2004

52. Storms WW: Review of exercise-induced asthma. Med Sci Sports Exerc 2003;35(9):1464-1470

53. National Asthma Education and Prevention Program, Expert panel report: guidelines for the diagnosis and management of asthma: update on selected topics 2002. Bethesda, MD, National Institutes of Health, 2003. NIH Publication No 02-5074

54. Storms WW: Exercise-induced asthma: diagnosis and treatment for the recreational or elite athlete. Med Sci Sports Exerc 1999;31(1 suppl):S33-S38

55. Feinstein RA, LaRussa J, Wang-Dohlman A, et al: Screening adolescent athletes for exercise-induced asthma. Clin J Sport Med 1996;6(2):119-123

56. Johansson H, Foucard T, Pettersson LG: Exercise tests in large groups of children are not a suitable screening procedure for undiagnosed asthma. Allergy 1997;52(11):1128-1132

57. American College of Allergy, Asthma and Immunology: Asthma Disease Management Resource Manual. Available at http://allergy.mcg.edu/physicians/manual/manual.html. Accessed August 9, 2004

58. Becker JM, Rogers J, Rossini G, et al: Asthma deaths during sports: a report of a 7-year experience. J Allergy Clin Immunol 2004;113(2):264-267

59. American Academy of Pediatrics Committee on Sports Medicine and Fitness: Medical conditions affecting sports participation. Pediatrics 2001;107(5):1205-1209

60. Vincent MT, Celestin N, Hussain AN: Pharyngitis. Am Fam Physician 2004;69(6):1465-1470

61. Middleton DB: Pharyngitis. Prim Care 1996;23(4):719-739

62. The American Academy of Family Physicians Web site: http://familydoctor.org/

63. MacKnight JM: Infectious mononucleosis: ensuring a safe return to sport. Phys Sportsmed 2002;30(1):27-41

64. The National Collegiate Athletic Association Committee on Competitive Safeguards and Medical Aspects of Sports: NCAA Injury Surveillance System (ISS). Available at http://www1.ncaa.org/membership/ed_outreach/health-safety/iss/index.html. Accessed August 6, 2004

65. NCAA Wrestling 2004 Rules and Interpretations. Indianapolis, IN, National Collegiate Athletic Association, August 2003. ISSN #0736-511X

66. Skin infections in wrestling: sports medicine guidelines, in Schluep C (ed): NCAA Sports Medicine Handbook 2003-2004, ed 16. Indianapolis, IN, National Collegiate Athletic Association, August 2003, p 21

67. Anderson BJ: The epidemiology and clinical analysis of several outbreaks of herpes gladiatorum. Med Sci Sports Exerc 2003;35(11):1809-1814

68. Organizations plan to reduce herpes gladiatorum outbreaks through earlier diagnosis and treatment. American College of Sports Medicine news release, November 17, 2003. Available at http//www.acsm.org. Accessed August 9, 2004

69. Howe WB: Preventing infectious disease in sports. Phys Sportsmed 2003;31(2):23-29

70. Kohl TD, Lisney M: Tinea gladiatorum: wrestling's emerging foe. Sports Med 2000;29(6):439-447

71. Adams BB: Tinea corporis gladiatorum. J Am Acad Dermatol 2002;47(2):286-290

72. Beck CK: Infectious diseases in sports. Med Sci Sports Exerc 2000;32(7 suppl):S431-S438

73. Barrett TW, Moran GJ: Update on emerging infections: news from the Centers for Disease Control and Prevention. Methicillin-resistant Staphylococcus aureus infections among competitive sports participants—Colorado, Indiana, Pennsylvania, and Los Angeles County, 2000-2003. Ann Emerg Med 2004;43(1);43-45

74. Aubrey M, Cantu R, Dvorak J, et al: Summary and agreement statement of the First International Conference on Concussion in Sport, Vienna 2001. Phys Sportsmed 2002;30(3):57-63

75. Kushner DS: Concussion in sports: minimizing the risk for complications. Am Fam Physician 2001;64(6):1007-1014

76. The American Academy of Neurology: Practice parameter: the management of concussion in sports (summary statement). Report of the Quality Standards Subcommittee. Neurology 1997;48(3):581-585

77. Concussion and second impact syndrome: sports medicine guidelines, in Schluep C (ed): NCAA Sports Medicine Handbook 2003-2004, ed 16. Indianapolis, IN, National Collegiate Athletic Association, August 2003, p 54

78. Kelly JP, Rosenberg JH: The development of guidelines for the management of concussion in sports. J Head Trauma Rehabil 1998;13(2):53-65

79. Rabadi MH, Jordon BD. The cumulative effect of repetitive concussion in sports. Clin J Sport Med 2001;11(3):194-198

80. Wojtys EM, Hovda D, Landry G, et al: Current concepts: concussion in sports. Am J Sports Med 1999;27(5):676-687

81. McCrea M, Kelly JP, Kluge J, et al: Standardized assessment of concussion in football players. Neurology 1997;48(3):586-588

82. Maddocks DL, Dicker GD, Saling MM: The assessment of orientation following concussion in athletes. Clin J Sport Med 1995;5(1):32-35

83. McCrory P: Does second impact syndrome exist? Clin J Sport Med 2001;11(3):144-149

84. Kushner D: Mild traumatic brain injury: toward understanding manifestations and treatment. Arch Intern Med 1998;158(15):1617-1624

85. Cantu RC: Guidelines for return to contact sports after a cerebral concussion. Phys Sportsmed 1986;14(10):75-83

86. Colorado Medical Society Sports Medicine Committee: Guidelines for the management of concussion in sports. Denver, Colorado Medical Society, 1991

87. Committee on Quality Improvement, American Academy of Pediatrics, Commission on Clinical Policies and Research, American Academy of Family Physicians: The management of minor closed head injury in children. Pediatrics 1999;104(6):1407-1415

88. Johnston KM, McCory P, Mohtadi NG, et al: Evidence-based review of sport-related concussion: clinical science. Clin J Sport Med 2001;11(3):150-159

89. Brain Injury Association of America, 8201 Greensboro Drive, Suite 611, McLean, Virginia 22102.. Web site: http://biausa.org/pages/home.html. Accessed August 9, 2004

90. Dubow JS, Kelly JP: Epilepsy in sports and recreation. Sports Med 2003;33(7):499-516

91. Hirtz D, Berg A, Bettis D, et al: Practice parameter: treatment of the child with a first unprovoked seizure: report of the Quality Standards Subcommittee of the American Academy of Neurology and the Practice Committee of the Child Neurology Society. Neurology 2003;60(2):166-175

92. Lewis DW, Ashwal S, Dahl G, et al: Practice parameter: evaluation of children and adolescents with recurrent headaches: report of the Quality Standards Subcommittee of the American Academy of Neurology and the Practice Committee of the Child Neurology Society. Neurology 2002;59(4):490-498

93. McCrory P: Recognizing exercise-related headache. Phys Sportsmed 1997;25(2):33-43

94. Sallis RE, Jones K, Knopp W: Burners: offensive strategy for an underreported injury. Phys Sportsmed 1992;20(11):47-55

95. Castro FP Jr: Stingers, cervical cord neuropraxia, and stenosis. Clin Sports Med 2003;22(3):483-492

96. Meyer SA, Schulte KR, Callaghan JJ, et al: Cervical spinal stenosis and stingers in collegiate football players. Am J Sports Med 1994;22(2):158-166

97. Shannon B, Klimkiewicz JJ: Cervical burners in the athlete. Clin Sports Med 2002;21(1):29-35

98. Aldridge JW, Bruno RJ, Strauch RJ, et al: Nerve entrapment in athletes. Clin Sports Med 2001;20(1):95-122

99. Bergfeld JA, Hershman ER, Wilbourn AJ: Brachial plexus injury in sports: a five-year follow-up. Orthop Trans 1988;12:743-744

100. Speer KP, Bassett FH 3rd: The prolonged burner syndrome. Am J Sports Med 1990;18(6):591-594

101. Levitz CL, Reilly PJ, Torg JS: The pathomechanics of chronic, recurrent cervical nerve root neurapraxia: the chronic burner syndrome. Am J Sports Med 1997; 25(1):73-76

102. Weinberg J, Rokito S, Silber JS: Etiology, treatment, and prevention of athletic "stingers". Clin Sports Med 2003; 22(3):493-500, viii

103. Feinberg JH: Burners and stingers. Phys Med Rehabil Clin N Am 2000;11(4):771-784

104. Torg JS: Epidemiology, pathomechanics, and prevention of athletic injuries to the cervical spine. Med Sci Sports Ex 1985; 17(3):295-303

105. Cross KM, Serenelli C: Training and equipment to prevent athletic head and neck injuries. Clin Sports Med 2003;22 (3):639-667

106. "Burners" (Brachial Plexus Injuries): sports medicine guidelines, in Schluep C (ed): NCAA Sports Medicine Handbook 2003-2004, ed 16. Indianapolis, IN, National Collegiate Athletic Association, August 2003, p 51

107. National Center for Catastrophic Sport Injury Research: Eighteenth Annual Report, Fall 1982-Spring 2000, Chapel Hill, NC, University of North Carolina, 2000 Available at http://www.unc.edu/depts/nccsi/allsport.htm. Accessed August 9, 2004

108. Koffler KM, Kelly JD 4th: Neurovascular trauma in athletes. Orthop Clin N Am 2002;33(3):523-534, vi

109. Barrow MW, Clark KA: Heat-related illnesses. Am Fam Physician 1998;58(3):749-759

110. Inter-Association Task Force on Exertional Heat Illness Consensus Statement. National Athletic Trainers Association, June 2003. Available at http://www.nata.org/ industryresources/heatillnessconcensusstatement.pdf. Accessed August 9, 2004

111. Prevention of heat illness: sports medicine guidelines, in Schluep C (ed): NCAA Sports Medicine Handbook 2003-2004, ed 16. Indianapolis, IN, National Collegiate Athletic Association, August 2003, p 22

112. American Academy of Pediatrics Committee on Sports Medicine and Fitness: Climatic heat stress and the exercising child and adolescent. Pediatrics 2000;106(1 pt 1): 158-159

113. Kulka TJ, Kenney WL: Heat balance limits in football uniforms: how different uniform ensembles alter the equation. Phys Sportsmed 2002;30(7):29-39

114. Pretzlaff RK: Death of an adolescent athlete with sickle cell trait caused by exertional heat stroke. Pediatr Crit Care Med 2002;3(3):308-310

115. Kark JA, Posey DM, Schumacher HR, et al: Sickle-cell trait as a risk factor for sudden death in physical training. N Engl J Med 1987;317(13):781-787

116. Drehner D, Neuhauser KM, Neuhauser TS, et al: Death among U.S. Air Force basic trainees: 1956 to 1996. Mil Med 1999;164(12):841-847

117. American Academy of Orthopaedic Surgeons and American Academy of Pediatrics, Sullivan JA, Anderson SJ, (eds): Care of the Young Athlete: Practical guide to preparation, participation, and injury treatment in childhood athletics. Elk Grove Village, IL, American Academy of Pediatrics, 2000

118. Ramirez A , Hartley LH, Rhodes D, et al: Morphological features of red blood cells in subjects with sickle cell trait: changes during exercise. Arch Intern Med 1976;136(9):1064-1066

119. Kerle KK, Nishimura KD: Exertional collapse and sudden death associated with sickle cell trait. Am Fam Physician 1996;54(1):237-240

120. American Academy of Pediatrics Committee on Practice and Ambulatory Medicine, Section on Ophthalmology: Eye examination and vision screening in infants, children, and young adults.. Pediatrics 1996;98(1):153-157

121. Sports and Recreational Eye Injuries. US Consumer Product Safety Commission, 2000

122. American Academy of Pediatrics Committee on Sports Medicine and Fitness: Protective eyewear for young athletes. Pediatrics 2004;113(3):619-622

123. Sports medicine: protective equipment required for girls lacrosse. National Federation of State High School Associations news release, July 10, 2003. Available at http://www.nfhs.org/scriptcontent/va_custom/va_cm/cont entpagedisplay.cfm?content_id=213. Accessed August 10, 2004

124. Web site for USA Hockey: http://www.usahockey.com. Accessed August 9, 2004

125. Jeffers JB: An on-going tragedy: pediatric sports-related eye injuries. Semin Opthalmol 1990;5:216-223

126. Larrison WI, Hersh PS, Kunzweiler T, et al: Sports-related ocular trauma. Ophthalmology 1990;97(10):1265-1269

127. Strahlman E, Sommer A: The epidemiology of sports-related ocular trauma. Int Ophthalmol Clin 1988;28(3): 199-202

128. Tanner SM: Preparticipation examination targeted for the female athlete. Clin Sports Med 1994:13(2):337-353

129. Johnson C, Powers PS, Dick R: Athletes and eating disorders: the National Collegiate Athletic Association study. Int J Eat Disord 1999;26(2):179-188

130. Web site for Academy for Eating Disorders: www.aedweb.org. Accessed August 9, 2004

131. Garrow JS, Webster J: Quetelet's index (W/H2) as a measure of fatness. Int J Obes 1985;9(2):147-153

132. Web site for Centers for Disease Control and Prevention: http://www.cdc.gov. Accessed August 9, 2004

133. American Diabetes Association: Type 2 diabetes in children and adolescents. Pediatrics 2000;105(3 pt 1):671-680

134. American Academy of Pediatrics Committee on Sports Medicine and Fitness: Promotion of healthy weight-control practices in young athletes. Pediatrics. 1996;97(5):752-753

135. Himes JH, Dietz WH: Guidelines for overweight in adolescent preventive services: recommendations from an expert committee. The Expert Committee on Clinical Guidelines for Overweight in Adolescent Preventive Services. Am J Clin Nutr 1994;59(2):307-316

136. The Surgeon General's call to action to prevent and decrease overweight and obesity 2001. Rockville, MD, US Department of Health and Human Services, Public Health Service, Office of the Surgeon General, 2001. Available at http://surgeongeneral.gov.library. Accessed August 9, 2004

137. Jiménez CE: Preparing active patients for international travel. Phys Sportsmed 2003;31(10):27-35

138. US Department of Health and Human Services, Centers for Disease Control and Prevention: Assessing Health Risk Behaviors Among Young People: Youth Rsk Behavior Surveillance System, 2004. Available at http://www.cdc.gov/ yrbss. Accessed August 9, 2004

139. US Department of Health and Human Services: Healthy People 2010: Understanding and Improving Health, ed 2. Pittsburg, US Government Printing Office, November 2000. Publication number 017-001-00543-6. Available at http:// www.health.gov/healthypeople. Accessed August 9, 2004

140. National Institute of Mental Health, US Department of Health and Human Services: Suicide facts and statistics. Available at http://www.nimh.nih.gov/suicideprevention/ suifact.cfm. Accessed August 9, 2004

141. US Department of Health and Human Services, Centers for Disease Control and Prevention: Youth Risk Behavior

Surveillance System (YRBSS) National Youth Risk Behavior Survey 1991-2003: Trends in the prevalence of selected risk behaviors. Available at http://www.cdc.gov/yrbss. Accessed August 9, 2004

142. Escher SA, Tucker AM, Lundin TM, et al: Smokeless tobacco, reaction time, and strength in athletes. Med Sci Sports and Exerc 1998;30(10):1548-1551

143. National Association of State High School Associations: The coaches code of ethics. Available at http://www.nfhs.org/scriptcontent/va_Custom/va_cm/contentpagedisplay.cfm?content_id=253. Accessed August 9, 2004

144. Institutional alcohol, tobacco, and other drug education programs: sports medicine guidelines, in Schluep C (ed): NCAA Sports Medicine Handbook 2003-2004, ed 16. Indianapolis, IN, National Collegiate Athletic Association, August 2003, p 15

145. Web site for World Anti-Doping Agency: http://www.wada-ama.org. Accessed August 9, 2004

146. Web site for United States Anti-Doping Agency: http://www.usantidoping.org. Accessed August 9, 2004

147. American College of Sports Medicine position stand on the use of alcohol in sports. Med Sci Sports Exerc 1982;14(6):ix-xi

148. Web site for 2004 US Olympic team: http://www.olympic-usa.org. Accessed August 9, 2004

149. National Collegiate Athletic Association: NCAA Banned-Drug Classes 2004-2005. Available at http://www1.ncaa.org/membership/ed_outreach/healthsafety/drug_testing/banned_drug_classes.pdf. Accessed August 9, 2004

150. Zickler, Patrick: Annual survey finds increasing teen use of ecstasy, steroids. National Institute of Drug Abuse, NIDA Notes, May 2001, vol 16, no 2

151. American Academy of Pediatrics Committee on Sports Medicine and Fitness: Adolescents and anabolic steroids: a subject review. Pediatrics 1997;99(6):904-908

152. American College of Sports Medicine position stand on the use of anabolic-androgenic steroids in sports. Med Sci Sports Exerc 1987;19(5):534-539

153. US Food and Drug Administration: Dietary Supplement Health and Education Act of 1994, Public Law 103-417. Available at http://www.fda.gov/opacom/laws/dshea.html. Accessed August 10, 2004

154. United States Anti-Doping Agency: 2004 Guide to prohibited substances and prohibited methods of doping. Available at: http://www.usantidoping.org/athletes/downloads.aspx. Accessed August 9, 2004

155. World Anti-Doping Agency: List of prohibited substances and methods: 2004 prohibited list. Available at www.wada-ama.org/en/t3.asp?p=41510. Accessed August 9, 2004

Chapter 6

THE PPE PHYSICAL EXAMINATION

The physical examination in the PPE is a screening tool emphasizing the areas of greatest concern in sports participation and areas identified as problems in the history. It is meant to identify individuals who may be at a cardiovascular or neurologic high risk (associated with severe disability or death) during sports participation.[1] Also, athletes who may have health problems should be referred to their primary care physician or to a specialist if they have no primary care provider.

Table 15 lists the components of the physical examination. Males should be dressed in shorts and females in shorts and tank tops to facilitate an adequate examination. The form on page 94 can be used for the complete or interim (page 8) PPE physical exam.

◤ HEIGHT AND WEIGHT

Height and weight are measured and recorded. Extremely thin individuals may warrant questioning about recent weight loss, eating habits, or body image. Referral to their primary care physician (or specialist if they have no primary care physician) for further evaluation is indicated if an eating disorder (eg, anorexia or bulimia) or growth disturbance is suspected. Obese and overweight athletes can be referred for counseling on diet, exercise, and behavior modification for weight control.

Body composition is one part of a person's overall physical fitness (see, "What Is the Body Mass Index?" on the next page). The others are cardiovascular endurance, muscle strength, and flexibility. The first two parts are linked with the risk of heart and blood vessel disease. Obesity is now recognized as a major, independent risk factor for heart disease.

Obesity is the most prevalent nutritional disorder among children and adolescents in the United States. Obesity in childhood and adolescence represents a serious concern and a challenge to the medical and lay communities.[2] Major impacts include effects on blood pressure, intermediary metabolism, respiratory function, psychological well-being, social adaptation, and educational performance.[3]

Obesity is particularly dangerous for younger adults. Severely obese white men, 20 to 30 years old, live about 13 fewer years than others in the general population.[4] Severely obese white women can expect to live 8 fewer years than their nonobese counterparts. Obesity also has a profound effect on the lifespan of younger blacks. Obese black men, 20 to 30 years old, lose about 20 years, and obese black women lose about 5 years of life, even after adjusting the data for smoking.[4]

Freemark[3] states that, using BMI criteria, national surveys demonstrate that 21% to 24% of American children and adolescents are overweight and that 10%

Table 15 Standard Components of the Preparticipation Physical Examination

Height
Weight
Eyes
　Visual acuity (Snellen chart)
　Differences in pupil size
Oral Cavity
Ears
Nose
Lungs
Cardiovascular System
　Blood pressure
　Pulses (radial, femoral)
　Heart (rate, rhythm, murmurs)
Abdomen
　Masses
　Tenderness
　Organomegaly
Genitalia (Males Only)
　Single or undescended testicle
　Testicular mass
　Hernia
Skin
　Rashes
　Lesions
Musculoskeletal System
　Contour, range of motion, stability, and symmetry of neck, back, shoulder/arm, elbow/forearm, wrist/hand, hip/thigh, knee, leg/ankle, foot

WHAT IS THE BODY MASS INDEX?

Measuring body mass index (BMI) is the easiest way to measure a person's body composition (a component of a person's overall physical fitness).[1] The BMI is the calculated derived ratio of height and weight and is used differently in children than in adults. In a child, BMI is used to assess underweight, overweight, and risk for overweight (table A). A child's body fatness changes with age and growth. Additionally, boys' and girls' body fatness change differently as they mature. Thus, BMI for children, also referred to as BMI-for-age, is gender and age specific. BMI-for-age is plotted on gender-specific growth charts provided by the CDC. These charts are used for children and teens 2 to 20 years old (www.cdc.gov/growthcharts).

REFERENCE

1. The Practical Guide Identification, Evaluation, and Treatment of Overweight and Obesity in Adults; U.S. Department of Health and Human Services, Public Health Service, National Institutes of Health National Heart, Lung, and Blood Institute, NIH Publication No. 00-4084, October 2000

Table A	BMI-for-Age Categories for Those 2 to 20 Years Old

Weight Category	BMI-for-Age
Underweight	<5th percentile
At risk of overweight	85th-95th percentile
Overweight	≥ 95th percentile

Source: www.cdc.gov/nccdphp/dnpa/bmi/bmi-for-age.htm.

to 11% are obese. He further states that the prevalence of US children and adolescents whose BMI is at or above the 85th percentile (overweight or at risk of becoming overweight, according to the CDC) has increased by 50% to 60% in a single generation, while the prevalence of obesity has doubled. In addition, the prevalence of obesity in American Indians, Hawaiians, Hispanics, and blacks is 10% to 40% higher than that in whites. Finally, preliminary research shows that children with a BMI at the 95th percentile or greater at 18 years of age will have a 66% to 78% greater risk of being overweight at age 35.[3]

Determination of body composition with skinfold calipers or other devices is an optional component of the PPE. It may allow estimation of an ideal weight range in sports requiring weight control, such as wrestling. Additionally, calipers may more accurately measure body composition of the thin athletes and more accurately represent muscular athletes, who frequently have a falsely high BMI and may falsely be considered obese. It is difficult, however, to predict the exact ideal percentage of body fat for a participant in a given sport. Those with abnormal BMI (verified by body composition assessment) should be referred for follow-up.

◤ HEAD, EYES, EARS, NOSE, AND THROAT (HEENT)

Visual acuity, measured with a standard Snellen eye chart, should be 20/40 or better in each eye, with or without corrective lenses. Athletes who have 1 eye missing, best corrected vision poorer than 20/40 in either eye, or a history of significant eye injury or surgery will need appropriate eye protection if they wish to participate in sports that have a high risk of eye injury (see page 70). If the athlete already has protective eyewear, this should be checked to ensure that it is in good condition and is of the appropriate type (see page 71). All athletes should be reminded about appropriate eye protection for their respective sports.

The pupils should be examined for anisocoria (unequal size). Although many people have a slight difference in pupil size (physiologic anisocoria), a marked difference in pupil size occasionally may be noted in otherwise normal eyes. It is imperative to be aware of baseline anisocoria when evaluating a head injury. Communicating this information to the athletic trainer and/or coach is important if the examination record is not present at all practices and games.

The remainder of the HEENT examination assesses general well-being of these areas. The clinician should be alert to oral ulcers, gingival atrophy, and decreased enamel seen in those with disordered eating behaviors, especially bulimia; leukoplakia seen in smokeless tobacco users; a high-arched palate (minor diagnostic criteria)[5] in athletes with other characteristics of Marfan syndrome (see the "Musculoskeletal System" section [page 51] for other diagnostic criteria and table 6 for complete diagnostic criteria [page 23]); corrective braces on the teeth that may require use of a mouth guard to prevent laceration from oral trauma; scarring of the tympanic membrane or auditory canals related to prior tympanostomy tube or prior infection (if indicated, a hearing screen should be performed); perforated tympanic membranes in athletes competing in water sports who would need protective earplugs; and adenopathy that may suggest malignancy or infection. Nasal polyps or a deviated septum do not affect clearance but can be identified and the patient referred for further evaluation and possible treatment.

◣ CARDIOVASCULAR SYSTEM

Blood pressure should be measured with an appropriately sized cuff (large athletes may require a thigh cuff for the arm) and the measurement recorded. If blood pressure is initially elevated, the athlete should sit quietly for 5 minutes before repeating the measurements. If necessary, repeat the measurements a third time after the athlete lies down and rests for 10 to 15 minutes. If the athlete's blood pressure is still elevated according to the criteria in tables 16 and 17,[6,7] the athlete should be questioned about the use of stimulants (eg, caffeine, nicotine, ephedrine). The athlete should be referred for further evaluation and treatment, and clearance may be withheld or modified.

Table 16 — Classification of Hypertension in Children and Adolescents*

Blood Pressure Classification	Systolic and Diastolic Blood Pressure Measurement†
Normal	< 90th percentile for age, sex, and height
High normal	90th-95th percentile for age, sex, and height
Hypertension	> 95th-99th percentile for age, sex, and height
Severe hypertension	> 99th percentile for age, sex, and height

*Charts for classification by age, sex, and height percentile can be found at http://www.nhlbi.nih.gov/guidelines/hypertension/child_tbl.htm.
†On repeated measurement.

Sources: (1) National High Blood Pressure Education Program. Update on the 1987 Task Force Report on High Blood Pressure in Children and Adolescents: A working group report the the National High Blood Pressure Education Program. National High Blood Pressure Education Working Group on Hypertension Control in Children and Adolescents. Pediatrics 1996;98(pt 1):649-658; (2) http://www.nhlbi.nih.gov/guidelines/hypertension/child_tbl.htm.

Table 17 — Classification of Hypertension in Adults

Blood Pressure Classification*	Systolic Blood Pressure (mm Hg)†	Diastolic Blood Pressure (mm Hg)†
Normal	< 120	and < 80
Prehypertension	120-139	or 80-89
Stage 1 Hypertension	140-159	or 90-99
Stage 2 Hypertension	≥ 160	or ≥ 100

*Classification determined by highest systolic or diastolic blood pressure category.
†Based on the average of 2 or more properly measured, seated readings on each of 2 or more office visits.

Source: The Seventh Report of the Joint National Committee on Prevention, Detection, Evaluation, and Treatment of High Blood Pressure (JNC 7). US Dept of Health and Human Services, National Institutes of Health, National Heart, Lung, and Blood Institute, 2003. Available at http://www.nhlbi.nih.gov/guidelines/hypertension/.

Palpation of the radial pulse is usually adequate to determine whether heart rate and rhythm are regular. Simultaneous palpation of the radial and femoral pulses is a screen for coarctation of the aorta.

Auscultation of the heart should be performed with the athlete in the supine and sitting or standing positions.[8] Standing is preferred to sitting, because the diagnostic murmur of hypertrophic cardiomyopathy (HCM) tends to be louder when the patient is standing; however, if no murmur is present as the athlete sits, there is little reason to have the athlete stand. Particular attention should be paid to the presence and character of any murmurs, the timing of murmurs in relation to S_1 and S_2, extra heart sounds (S_3, S_4), and clicks. Auscultatory effects of mitral valve prolapse include a midsystolic click and sometimes a late-systolic murmur (table 18).[9]

Various maneuvers, such as squat-to-stand, deep inspiration, or Valsalva's maneuver, can help clarify murmur type. Squatting increases venous return to the heart, which in turn increases left ventricular blood volume, stroke volume, and systemic vascular resistance. Returning to a standing position reverses these changes. Valsalva's maneuver has the opposite effects by decreasing venous return to the heart. With HCM, therefore, squatting decreases the outflow obstruction and decreases the intensity of the murmur, while Valsalva's maneuver increases the obstruction and increases the murmur. The harsh, systolic murmur of aortic stenosis, on the other hand, increases with squatting and decreases with Valsalva's maneuver. The intensity of innocent murmurs also increases with

Table 18 — Effects of Physiologic Maneuvers on Auscultatory Events

Maneuver	Major Physiologic Effects	Useful Auscultatory Changes
Respiration	⇑Venous return with inspiration	⇑Right heart murmurs and gallops with inspiration; splitting of S_2
Valsalva (initial ⇑ BP, phase 1; followed by ⇓ BP, phase 2)	⇓ BP, venous return, LV size (phase 2)	⇑HCM ⇓AS, MR MVP click earlier in systole, murmur prolongs
Standing	⇓Venous return	⇑HCM; ⇓AS, MR; MVP click earlier in systole, murmur prolongs
Squatting	⇑Venous return, systemic vascular resistance, LV size	⇑AS, MR, AI: ⇓HCM; MVP click delayed, murmur shortens
Isometric exercise (eg, handgrip)	⇑ Arterial pressure, cardiac output	⇑MR, AI, MS ⇓AS, HCM
Post PVC or prolonged R-R interval	⇑Ventricular filling, contractility	⇑AS; little change in MR
Amyl nitrate	⇓ Arterial pressure, LV size ⇑ Cardiac output	⇑HCM, AS, MS ⇓AI, MR, Austin Flint murmur; MVP click earlier in systole, murmur prolongs
Phenylephrine	⇑ Arterial pressure, LV size ⇓ Cardiac output	⇑ MR, AI; ⇓ AS, HCM; MVP click delayed, murmur shortens

⇑ = increased intensity; ⇓ = decreased intensity; AI = aortic insufficiency; AS = aortic stenosis; BP = blood pressure; HCM = hypertrophic cardiomyopathy; LV = left ventricular; MR = mitral regurgitation; MS = mitral stenosis; MVP = mitral valve prolapse; PVC = premature ventricular contraction; R-R = interval between the R waves on an ECG

Reprinted with permission from Carpenter CJ, Griggs RC, Loscalzo J (eds): Cecil Essentials of Medicine, ed 6. Philadelphia, Saunders, 2004, p 43.

Table 19 — Classification of Heart Murmurs

Timing	Class	Description	Characteristic Lesions
Systolic	Ejection	Begins in early systole; may extend to mid or late systole; crescendo-decrescendo pattern; often harsh in quality	Valvular, supravalvular, and subvalvular aortic stenosis; HCM; pulmonic stenosis; aortic or pulmonary artery dilation; malformed but nonobstructive aortic valve; (transvalvular flow (eg, aortic rugurgitation, hyperkinetic states, ASD, physiologic flow murmur)
	Holo-systolic	Extends throughout systole; relatively uniform in intensity	MR; tricuspid regurgitation; ventricular septal defect
	Late	Variable onset and duration, often preceded by a nonejection click	MVP
Diastolic	Early	Begins with A2 or P2; decrescendo pattern with variable duration; often high-pitched, blowing	Aortic regurgitation
	Mid	Begins after S_2, often after an opening snap; low-pitched "rumble" heard best with bell of stethoscope	Mitral stenosis; tricuspid stenosis; ⇧ flow across AV valves (eg, MR, tricuspid regurgitation, ASD)
	Late	Presystolic accentuation of mid-diastolic murmur	Mitral stenosis; tricuspid stenosis
Continuous		Systolic and diastolic components; "machinery" murmurs	Patent ductus aerteriosus; coronary AV fistula; ruptured sinus of Valsalva aneurysm into right atrium or ventricle; mammary souffle; venous hum

HCM = hypertrophic cardiomyopathy; ASD = atrial septal defect; MR = mitral regurgitation; MVP = mitral valve prolapse; AV = atrioventricular

Reprinted with permission from Carpenter CJ, Griggs RC, Loscalzo J (eds): Cecil Essentials of Medicine, ed 6. Philadelphia, Saunders, 2004, p 45.

squatting and decreases with Valsalva's maneuver, but an innocent murmur can be distinguished from an aortic stenosis murmur by volume, location, duration, quality, and radiation (table 19).[9]

In short, murmurs in adolescents are common, but any systolic murmur grade 3/6 in severity or more (table 20),[9] any diastolic murmur, and any murmur that gets louder with Valsalva's maneuver or with standing should be further evaluated before an athlete is cleared to play. If there is any uncertainty about the nature of the murmur, any cardiac symptoms noted in the history, or any family history of sudden cardiac death, the athlete should be referred for further evaluation and/or appropriate treatment.

Also, it must be remembered that the physical examination and auscultation alone cannot detect all

Table 20 — Grading System for Intensity of Murmurs

Grade	Description
1	Barely audible murmur
2	Murmur of medium intensity
3	Loud murmur, no thrill
4	Loud murmur, with thrill
5	Very loud murmur; stethoscope must be on the chest to hear it; may be heard posteriorly
6	Murmur audible with stethoscope off the chest

Reprinted with permission from Carpenter CJ, Griggs RC, Loscalzo J (eds): Cecil Essentials of Medicine, ed 6. Philadelphia, Saunders, 2004, p 43.

cases or types of heart disease,[10] and the appropriate screening questions are embedded in the PPE form. As the AHA states, "A complete and careful personal and family history and physical examination designed to identify, or raise suspicion of, those cardiovascular lesions known to cause sudden death or disease progression in young athletes is the best available and most practical approach to screening populations of competitive sports participants, regardless of age."[8]

Arrhythmias found on examination may require further evaluation, which may include ECG, Holter monitoring, exercise stress testing, and/or additional studies to determine their specific nature. Historically, during ECG evaluation, the disappearance of irregular beats with exercise usually indicates a benign condition in a structurally normal heart. If there are multifocal premature ventricular contractions, doublets, or triplets upon ECG, the athlete should be examined by a cardiologist.

In athletes who may have structural heart disease, the standard evaluation generally includes a history and physical, 12-lead ECG, stress echocardiogram, and graded exercise test. Evaluation beyond these tests usually requires the expertise of an experienced cardiologist. The 26th Bethesda Conference guidelines[11] remain an excellent resource for the primary care physician concerning the cardiovascular workup and return-to-play recommendations, as is the AHA's recent consensus statement.[12]

◣ LUNGS

Pulmonary examination should reveal clear breath sounds. Pathologic findings, such as wheezes, rubs, prolonged expiratory phase, or significant cough with forced expiration, should be referred for further evaluation and/or appropriate treatment. If the athlete smells of tobacco, a discussion regarding tobacco use may be in order. A normal examination does not exclude EIA, and provocative testing may be needed at a follow-up visit if the history suggests that the athlete has a problem during or immediately after exercise.

◣ ABDOMEN

The abdomen examination should be performed with the athlete supine. The anterior superior iliac spines should be exposed to ensure adequate inspection and palpation of all four quadrants. Abdominal masses, tenderness, rigidity, or enlargement of the liver

or spleen requires further evaluation prior to clearance. Occasionally, an abnormal kidney may be identified by abdomen examination, again requiring further evaluation. The lower abdominal examination in the female athlete should be prefaced by a brief explanation of the reason for additional regional evaluation. This brief introduction will help establish rapport for an exam that is sensitive by nature. If necessary, a chaperone can be obtained at the athlete's discretion. The focus of the examination is to determine the presence of a palpable (gravid) uterus, but a more detailed pelvic examination should be performed by the athlete's primary care physician or a designated specialist.

◣ GENITALIA

The male genitourinary examination should begin with a brief description of and reason for the examination, again, to establish rapport. If necessary, a chaperone can be provided at the athlete's discretion. The focus of the examination is to determine the presence of both testicles, testicular irregularities or masses, and inguinal canal hernias or pain. Counseling concerning participation in contact-collision sports is required for athletes with unpaired or undescended testicles, as discussed on page 76. Inguinal hernias should be evaluated on an individual basis. Inguinal canal pain may indicate a "sports hernia."

Testicular cancer is the leading cause of cancer deaths in men 15 to 35 years of age. The PPE provides an opportunity to introduce the health maintenance practice of testicular self-examination. The examining physician can let the athlete know that his testicles feel normal, encourage self-examination, and advise the athlete to see his physician if there are abnormal findings on the current exam or with future exams.

The genitourinary examination in female athletes is not part of the PPE. If a pelvic exam is warranted on the basis of the athlete's medical history or physical exam, it should be scheduled for a separate time.

Tanner staging for assessing physical maturity has not been contributory in determining clearance and likely would be useful only if the athlete had a history of growth or menstrual abnormalities suggestive of endocrine disease. Therefore, *the author societies no longer recommend Tanner staging as a routine part of the PPE.*[13,14] However, Tanner staging may be useful in boys 11 to 17 years old as a guide to counseling on topics of growth and development, sport safety, and steroid use. It is easy to do as part of the physical exam, and the staging reminds the physician to think about the physically immature boy playing against more physically mature males in collision sports such as ice hockey, lacrosse, and football.

◤ SKIN

Whether in an office-based or multiple-examiner setting, the skin should be inspected at a consistent point in the physical examination. Attention should be given to acne, evidence of sun damage, rashes, infections, marks of illicit drug use, and infestations. These include eczema, impetigo, furuncles or carbuncles, herpes simplex lesions, molluscum contagiosum, fungal infections, scabies, and louse infestations.[15-17]

A thorough search for abnormal nevi is not possible within the limits of the PPE; however, suspicious nevi noted during the examination should be referred for further evaluation and/or treatment. These lesions should not preclude clearance for participation. Contagious rash, especially for herpes, precludes contact with other athletes until the infection is adequately treated.

◤ MUSCULOSKELETAL SYSTEM

The type and extent of the musculoskeletal examination appropriate for the PPE is a much-debated topic, and few studies are available to guide the clinician. Examiners need to determine which method best suits a given situation, depending on history of injury, musculoskeletal signs or symptoms, resources and time available, type of sport or activity in which the athlete will participate, and the level of expertise of the examiner.

The yield of any type of musculoskeletal examination is low in asymptomatic athletes who have no history of injury. In addition, history alone has been shown to be 92% sensitive in detecting significant musculoskeletal injuries.[18] Therefore, a reasonable approach is to use a general screening examination (at right) for asymptomatic athletes who have no previous injury. If the athlete has (1) a previous injury or (2) pain, joint instability, locking, weakness, atrophy, or other signs or symptoms detected by the general screening examination or the history, the general screen should be supplemented with relevant elements of the joint-specific examination (at right), or the ath-

lete should be referred to a specialist for evaluation.[19,20] Alternatively, when time and resources permit, it is also reasonable to perform the entire joint-specific examination instead of a general screening examination, or to perform a sport-specific examination (see page 58).[20] Finally, an overview of skeletal structure may reveal the reduced upper-to-lower-segment ratio or arm-span-to-height ratio greater than 1.05 as 1 of the 4 major diagnostic criteria for Marfan syndrome.[21]

General screening examination. General screens may be used to quickly assess joint range of motion, gross muscle strength, and muscle asymmetry, and to identify significant injuries.[19] The general screening examination described here (figure 1)[22,23] is an adaptation of the 14-point musculoskeletal screening examination discussed in the second edition of this monograph.[13]

In using the general screen, however, clinicians must be aware that it does not allow determination of a specific diagnosis or severity of musculoskeletal injury. For example, it does not assess the degree of instability of a shoulder with glenohumeral joint laxity, and it may not allow for detection of rotator cuff injuries. Also, if the history indicates past or current ankle injury or pain, and the patient is unable to perform the toe raise or demonstrates obvious asymmetric lateral ankle swelling, ankle instability should be evaluated by anterior drawer and talar tilt tests. Examiners must therefore supplement the general screening examination with relevant elements of the joint-specific examination when indicated by findings in the history or general screen, or they must refer the athlete to a specialist for evaluation.

Joint-specific testing. Assessing individual joints by inspection, palpation, and maneuvers well established in the literature is more definitive than the general screening examination. It may also be better suited than the sport-specific examination (see page 58) to multisport athletes. However, joint-specific examinations are more time-consuming than the general screen, may exceed the expertise of the examiner, and have a low yield in an asymptomatic athlete without a previous injury. The author societies, therefore, do not consider it necessary to perform the entire joint-specific examination for every athlete. Instead, portions of the examination are used as indicated by the history and findings on the general screen. However, because of its accuracy, some practitioners

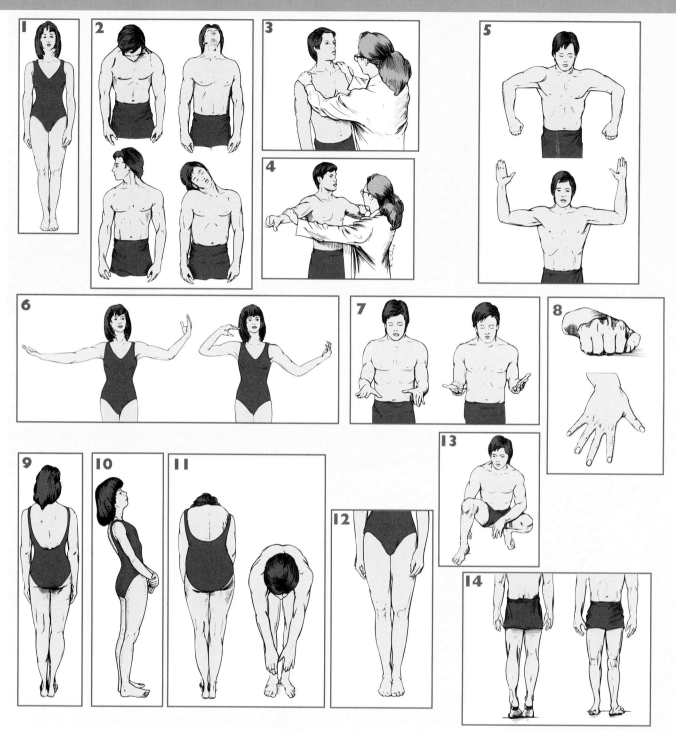

FIGURE 1. The general musculoskeletal screening examination consists of the following: **(1)** Inspection, athlete standing, facing toward examiner (symmetry of trunk, upper extremities); **(2)** Forward flexion, extension, rotation, lateral flexion of neck (range of motion, cervical spine); **(3)** Resisted shoulder shrug (strength, trapezius); **(4)** Resisted shoulder abduction (strength, deltoid); **(5)** Internal and external rotation of shoulder (range of motion, glenohumeral joint); **(6)** Extension and flexion of elbow (range of motion, elbow); **(7)** Pronation and supination of elbow (range of motion, elbow and wrist);

(8) Clench fist, then spread fingers (range of motion, hand and fingers); **(9)** Inspection, athlete facing away from examiner (symmetry of trunk, upper extremities); **(10)** Back extension, knees straight (spondylolysis/spondylolisthesis); **(11)** Back flexion with knees straight, facing toward and away from examiner (range of motion, thoracic and lumbosacral spine; spine curvature; hamstring flexibility); **(12)** Inspection of lower extremities, contraction of quadriceps muscles (alignment, symmetry); **(13)** "Duck walk" 4 steps (motion of hip, knee, and ankle; strength; balance); **(14)** Standing on toes, then on heels (symmetry, calf; strength; balance).

prefer to use the entire joint-specific examination as their primary evaluation tool during the musculoskeletal portion of the PPE.

The complete joint-specific screening examination includes inspection and range-of-motion testing of the neck, spine, shoulders, elbows, wrists, fingers, hips, knees, ankles, and feet. Stability of the shoulders, elbows, knees, and ankles is also assessed. Symmetry of joint appearance and motion should be noted.

If the joint-specific screening examination confirms a problem, a more thorough and focused examination with relevant diagnostic testing may be indicated prior to sports clearance. If the setting and examiner expertise allow, this exam may be done at the time of screening.

Spine. The cervical spine should be inspected for posture and alignment. Forward flexion of the neck should allow the chin to touch the manubrium, extension should allow skyward gaze, rotation should let the chin almost touch the clavicle in either direction, and the ears should approach the shoulders on lateral flexion. Any asymmetries or deficiencies should be noted.

Examination of the thoracolumbar spine focuses on appreciating deformities. The scapulae should be level, symmetric, and flat against the chest wall. Presence or absence of scoliosis should be observed, as well as the degree of kyphosis at the thoracic level and lordosis at the lumbar level. Presence of rotatory deformities should be noted as the athlete bends forward at the waist (figure 2); pain or restriction of motion on forward flexion may indicate lumbar disk disease. Back extension should also be assessed; pain may increase in the presence of spondylolysis, spondylolisthesis, or a strain.

Upper extremity. The shoulder examination begins with inspection for symmetry with the athlete standing. Range of motion in abduction (figure 3A), flexion (figure 3B), and internal and external rotation (figures 3C and 3D) are then assessed. The condition of the rotator cuff can be tested by several maneuvers, including the "empty can test" (figure 4A), manual resistance to internal and external rotation with the arm at the side (figure 4B), and by assessing for impingement symptoms (figures 4C and 4D). Deltoid strength is assessed by manual resistance to straight abduction. A screen for multidirectional instability includes subluxation tests in the anterior and posterior planes in the supine athlete (figures 5A through 5D), and in the inferior plane in the seated athlete (figure 5E).

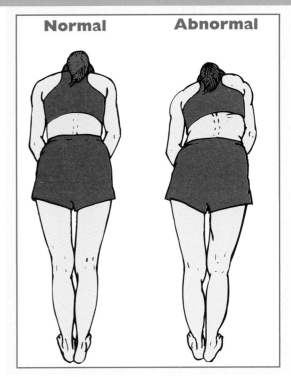

Figures 2-9. © 2005, Terry Boles

FIGURE 2. As part of the thoracolumbar spine examination, the athlete bends forward at the waist. The rotatory deformities of scoliosis, such as asymmetrical, prominent ribs, curvature of the spine, and/or an asymmetric waist, are accentuated in this position.

The elbow is observed for swelling, discoloration, and cubital angle (figure 6A). The elbow should extend fully and then flex to allow the athlete to touch the ipsilateral shoulder with the hand. Forearm motion is assessed by having the athlete pronate and supinate the forearms with the elbows bent 90° at his or her sides. The athlete should be able to turn the hand completely palm up and completely palm down.

In the throwing athlete, medial stability can be assessed by applying a valgus force to the elbow (figure 6B). The milking maneuver also assesses medial instability and is performed with the athlete's elbow flexed beyond 90° and the hand supinated. The examiner reaches behind the elbow being tested and grasps the affected MCL, applying a downward force. The test is considered positive if pain is noted over the MCL or if the joint opens medially. Direct comparison to the opposite arm is critical.

The hand and wrist are evaluated for symmetry. Wrists should palmar flex equally to about 80° and dorsiflex to 70° or more. There should be more ulnar deviation than radial deviation. The fingers should be

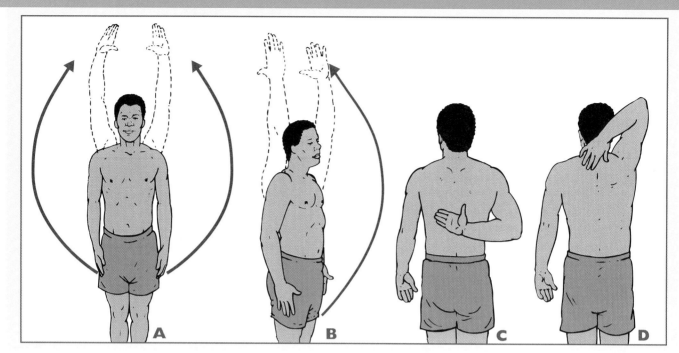

FIGURE 3. Shoulder range of motion is evaluated in 4 directions. In abduction (**A**) and forward flexion (**B**), the athlete should be able to reach completely overhead without excessive or asymmetric motion of the scapula; in internal rotation (**C**), the fingertips should reach approximately to the bottom of the opposite scapula; and in external rotation (**D**), the fingertips should approach the top of the opposite scapula.

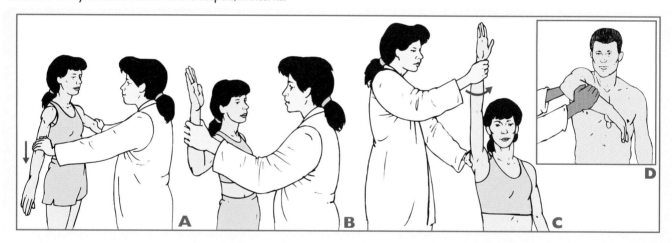

FIGURE 4. To assess rotator cuff function, the "empty can test" (**A**) can be used. The patient places both shoulders in 60° to 90° of abduction in the scapular plane, 30° forward flexion in the sagittal plane, full elbow extension, and forearm pronation (thumbs down); the examiner resists further abduction. Comparing manual resistance to further abduction in both internal and external rotation of the entire arm (**B**) helps distinguish biceps tendinopathy from rotator cuff pathology. Increased pain in external rotation as opposed to internal rotation should direct the examiner to further evaluate the rotator cuff, while the reverse is true in the case of biceps tendon pathology.* The Neer impingement test (**C**) involves fully abducting and forward flexing the shoulder and arm. An alternative exam for shoulder impingement, the Hawkin's test (**D**), involves forward flexion to 90° in the sagittal plane while the elbow is flexed to 90° and the shoulder is internally rotated. With internal shoulder rotation, the examiner notes whether there has been an exacerbation of shoulder pain. Localizing the exact site of the pain can help distinguish biceps tendinopathy or acromioclavicular pathology from rotator cuff pathology. If there is true outlet impingement, pain should localize to the anterior acromion of the shoulder and radiate laterally down the arm.

*Interestingly, 1 EMG study[24] suggests that forearm supination and greater than 45° of external humeral rotation (thumbs up) in 90° abduction better isolates the supraspinatus muscle from the other rotator cuff muscles. This would appear contrary to the examination described above. Whether or not this finding is clinically applicable requires further assessment.

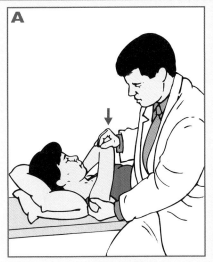

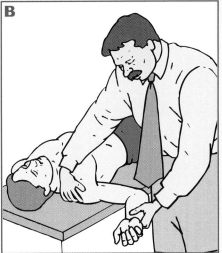

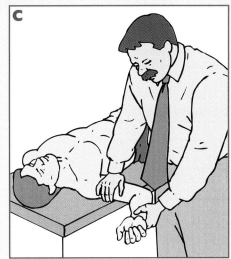

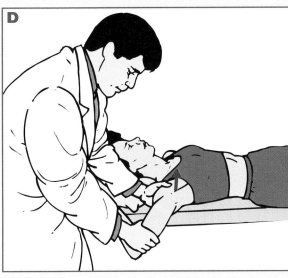

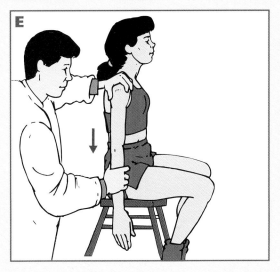

FIGURE 5. Multidirectional instability can be gauged by assessing glenohumeral motion in several planes. Posterior instability of the shoulder is assessed with the athlete supine by positioning the arm perpendicular to the table with the elbow bent, then applying pressure along the long axis of the arm **(A)**. The hand supporting the posterior shoulder palpates for excessive motion. When assessing shoulder internal rotation, it is important to stabilize the scapula by placing a hand against the scapular spine in the upright patient; in the supine patient, placing the shoulder firmly against the examination table can achieve the same goal. In the apprehension test **(B)**, which is used to assess for anterior instability, the examiner abducts the arm in the scapular plane and externally rotates the supine athlete's shoulder. It is important to look at the athlete's face while performing the maneuver to assess for visible signs of apprehension of a dislocation event. If apprehension is observed during the test, the relocation test **(C)** may be performed in the same position by applying a posteriorly directed force to the humeral head, reducing anterior translation of the humeral head. Relocation of the head will decrease the feeling of apprehension if instability is present. It is important to distinguish whether there is frank apprehension versus pain with this test. If the athlete experiences increasing pain with progressive external rotation of the humeral head, this suggests that the humeral head is subluxating anteriorly; secondary (internal) impingement of the rotator cuff is occurring, causing pain.[25] The augmentation test **(D)** is the reverse of the relocation test. An anteriorly directed force on the posterior proximal humerus, with the arm in 90° of abduction and maximal external rotation, will increase apprehension with anterior instability. The examiner's fingers should wrap around the humeral head anteriorly to prevent dislocation. When assessing the shoulder, it is important to examine the opposite arm to detect any asymmetry in degree of motion or instability between the shoulders. With the athlete seated **(E)**, inferior subluxation is confirmed by the presence of the sulcus sign— appearance of an indentation beneath the acromion with traction along the axis of the adducted arm. In the normal shoulder, there should be some inferior laxity with the arm at the side. However, as the arm is externally rotated with the arm maintained at the side, this laxity should correct as the rotator interval is placed in tension. Inferior subluxation that persists or is asymmetric to the opposite side suggests a tear of the rotator interval.

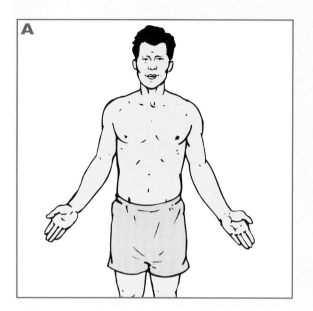

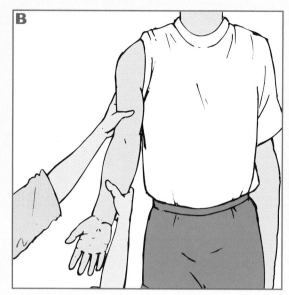

FIGURE 6. The normal carrying angle of the elbow is at least 15° valgus with the athlete standing and the palms forward **(A)**. An excessive valgus angle may indicate instability or a previous injury. In the throwing athlete, medial collateral ligament (MCL) instability should be assessed. This is accomplished by applying a valgus force to the elbow (with forearm pronation) at 25° to 30° of flexion while noting laxity and endpoint **(B)**. Placing the shoulder in maximal external rotation minimizes excessive humeral rotation, which may decrease the accuracy of medial stability testing.

able to close into a full fist, and each fingernail should point at the scaphoid bone with the fingers flexed across the palm. Intrinsic muscle function can be checked by having the athlete touch each fingertip with the thumb and spread and close the extended fingers.

Lower extremity. The hip examination begins with observation of the standing posture. Iliac crest height should be level, and the athlete should be able to stand on each foot without any tilting of the pelvis.

Hip range of motion can be assessed with the athlete lying supine. With the hip and the knee fully extended, the hip joint is rotated internally and externally (a "log roll" movement), and any asymmetry is noted. Symmetry of abduction and adduction should also be observed. Hip flexion should be beyond 90°, and the knees should come straight toward the chest; any external rotation indicates an intrinsic hip deformity. With the hip and knee flexed to 90°, the hip joint is rotated again (figure 7). Keeping the athlete's hip flexed 90° and extending the knee checks hamstring flexibility. The "popliteal angle" should be 0° to 10° but can vary based on patient age and sex.[26,27] The popliteal angle refers to the flexion angle of the knee created by tension in the hamstring tendons as the

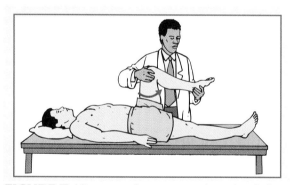

FIGURE 7. Hip range of motion is evaluated with the athlete supine. As part of the examination, the hip and knee are flexed to 90°, and the hip joint is rotated. A rotation arc of at least 60° should be observed. Pain or restriction of motion relative to the opposite side warrants further evaluation.

knee is extended while the hip is flexed.

With the athlete standing, inspection should reveal a normal leg-thigh valgus angulation of 12° or less in males and 18° or less in females. The patella should be observed for abnormal lateral subluxation or tilt or an excessively high position (patella alta) with the athlete seated.

The remainder of the knee examination should in-

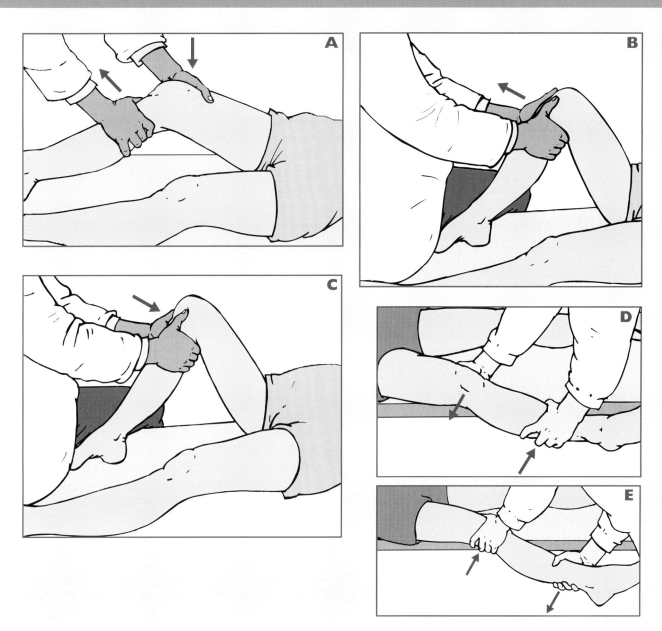

FIGURE 8. Several tests are used to assess ligamentous instability of the knee. For each test, the degree of excursion and the quality of the endpoint are noted and compared with the opposite side. The Lachman test **(A)** is the most sensitive means to assess anterior cruciate ligament (ACL) deficiencies.[28] The patient's knee is flexed approximately 20°, and the muscles are relaxed. The examiner stabilizes the femur with one hand while pulling the tibia anteriorly with the other hand. It is important to note how far the tibial tubercle translates anteriorly and whether there is a soft or firm endpoint at terminal translation. All findings should be compared with the opposite side. The anterior **(B)** and posterior **(C)** drawer tests can reveal ACL and posterior cruciate ligament (PCL) insufficiency, respectively. With the supine patient's knee bent 90°, the examiner sits on the patient's foot to stabilize it and grasps the proximal tibia. The hamstrings should be palpated to ensure they are relaxed. The examiner pulls the tibia anteriorly (anterior drawer test, B) and pushes it posteriorly (posterior drawer test, C) from the neutral position. With the anterior drawer test, lack of a firm endpoint and presence of excessive anterior tibial excursion suggest ACL insufficiency. With the posterior drawer test, the presence of excessive posterior tibial sag suggests PCL insufficiency. With an intact PCL, the tibia is positioned anterior to the femur with the knee in 90° of flexion. During the posterior drawer test, the examiner should palpate and quantify the change in anteromedial femoral-tibial step-off that occurs with and without a posteriorly directed force on the tibia. Varus **(D)** and valgus **(E)** stress tests gauge instability of the medial and lateral collateral ligaments of the knee. The athlete's knee is extended over the edge of the examination table and flexed to approximately 20°. One of the examiner's hands stabilizes the knee at the joint line, and varus and valgus stresses are applied to the tibia. Once again, comparison with the opposite limb is essential for these tests, given the normal range of variation in joint stability.

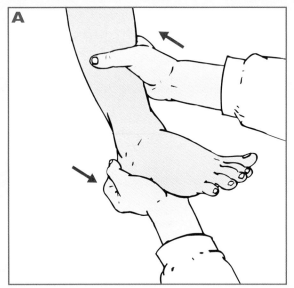

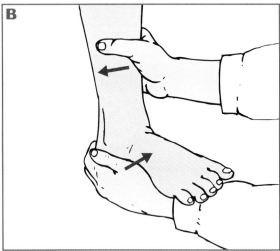

FIGURE 9. Two stress tests are used to assess instability of the ankle ligaments. For the anterior drawer test **(A)**, which demonstrates anterior subluxation, the examiner pulls the heel anteriorly while pushing posteriorly on the distal tibia. For the talar tilt test **(B)**, the examiner inverts the ankle by pushing laterally on the medial tibia and medially on the calcaneus. Excessive motion relative to the opposite side should trigger further evaluation.

volve both knees with the athlete supine. Each patella should be evaluated for hypermobility by translating the patella medially and laterally with the knee in approximately 20° of flexion; comparison with the opposite side should be made. Joint-line tenderness may indicate a meniscal tear. Any amount of knee effusion should be noted. Knee range of motion should be

from full extension to approximately 140° of flexion. Knee ligament stability tests include the Lachman test for anterior cruciate ligament deficiency (figure 8A); anterior and posterior drawer tests for anterior and posterior cruciate ligament insufficiencies, respectively (figures 8B and 8C); and varus and valgus stress tests for collateral ligament laxities (figures 8D and 8E).

The ankles are evaluated for normal appearance with the athlete first standing, then sitting. In the seated position, active dorsiflexion to 20° and plantar flexion to 40° should be present. With the knee extended, tightness in the Achilles tendon can be assessed by passively dorsiflexing the seated athlete's ankle while observing the lateral aspect of the leg and ankle. The ankle should dorsiflex 15° to 20° past neutral. Stress testing for ligament laxity includes the anterior drawer test for anterior subluxation (figure 9A) and the talar tilt test for lateral ligament stability (figure 9B).

On inspection of the foot, cavus or rigid flatfoot deformities should be noted. A supple flatfoot does not affect the athlete's performance but may be a risk factor for lower-extremity overuse problems such as medial tibial stress syndrome or patellofemoral pain. If the flatfoot is supple, the plantar arch will increase when the athlete stands on his or her toes. Toe deformities, including bunions, contractures, and pressure points indicated by calluses, may become painful in athletic footwear. Abnormalites associated with subtalar, midfoot, and forefoot problems should be further assessed through a formal gait and/or running study in an exercise physiology laboratory or similar facility.

Sport-specific examinations. Some sports medicine physicians advocate sport-specific physical examinations.[29,30] Such examinations focus on areas under particular stress (and therefore at higher risk for injury) in a given sport and include strength, endurance, and flexibility testing in addition to a more general orthopedic examination. For example, for swimmers and baseball pitchers, an examiner might measure shoulder internal and external rotation strength and endurance with isokinetic testing; for running and jumping athletes, the examiner might test knee flexion, extension, and strength with isokinetic testing and observe gait biomechanics on a treadmill.

Similarly, if there is evidence of hyperlaxity on examination, especially in the athlete engaged in overhead arm motions, growing evidence indicates that increased focus on the "joint(s) at risk" could be warranted.[31-33] For example, if an adolescent baseball pitcher or volleyball player comes in with limited, subtle, or frank shoulder complaints and has evidence of systemic laxity, such as hyperextension at the elbow, a thorough shoulder examination for labral pathology and shoulder subluxation should be performed. Another example is the adolescent soccer player with knee hyperextension and a history of knee problems. In this instance, a full ligamentous knee examination should be performed to assess for cruciate, collateral, and posterolateral corner knee instability. Additionally, referral may be indicated to assess for more serious conditions associated with generalized hypermobility (eg, Ehlers-Danlos syndrome, Marfan syndrome).

Although such precisely focused tests may reveal information that can improve performance and possibly prevent injury, these examinations are time-consuming and require more in-depth knowledge of individual sports than the joint-specific or general screening examination. When time, resources, and expertise al-

low, however, such examinations can supplement or replace the general screening examination and/or the joint-specific examination.

◤ NEUROLOGIC SYSTEM

In most cases, a normal musculoskeletal examination also implies normal motor neurologic function. However, additional neurologic testing may be required in certain situations. For example, in athletes who experience recurrent stingers or burners, an examination of the cervical spine and testing of upper-extremity strength and deep tendon reflexes are appropriate. An athlete who has had multiple or severe concussions needs a detailed history of these concussions, as described on page 28, but may also require examination of cranial nerves and motor, cerebellar, and cognitive function. Referral for a more comprehensive neurologic evaluation is warranted if any impairment is noted or if limited time and/or clinical expertise of the examining physician do not allow adequate neurologic evaluation during the PPE.

REFERENCES

1. Wingfield K, Matheson GO, Meeuwisse WH: Preparticipation evaluation: an evidence-based review. Clin J Sport Med 2004;14(3):109-122
2. Shephard RJ: Role of the physician in childhood obesity. Clin J Sport Med 2004;14(3):161-168
3. Freemark M: Obesity. emedicine: InstantAccess to the Minds of Medicine. Available at http://www.emedicine.com/ped/topic1699.htm#section-bibliography. Accessed July 19, 2004
4. Fontaine RR, Redden DT, Wang C, et al: Years of life lost due to obesity. JAMA 2003; 289(2):187-193
5. National Marfan Foundation: Marfan syndrome: an overview of related disorders. Available at http://www.marfan.org/nmf/GetSubContentRequestHandler.do?sub_menu_item_content_id=54&menu_item_id=42. Accessed July 19, 2004
6. National High Blood Pressure Education Working Group on Hypertension Control in Children and Adolescents: Update on the 1987 task force report on high blood pressure in children and adolescents: a working group report the the National High Blood Pressure Education Program. Pediatrics 1996;98(4 pt 1):649-658
7. The Seventh Report of the Joint National Committee on Prevention, Detection, Evaluation, and Treatment of High Blood Pressure (JNC 7). US Dept of Health and Human Services, National Institutes of Health, National Heart, Lung, and Blood Institute, 2003. Available at http://www.nhlbi.nih.gov/guidelines/hypertension/.Accessed July 19, 2004
8. Maron BJ, Thompson PD, Puffer JC, et al: Cardiovascular preparticipation screening of competitive athletes: a statement for health professionals from the Sudden Death Committee and Congenital Cardiac Defects Committee, American Heart Association. Circulation 1996;94(4):850-856
9. Carpenter CJ, Griggs RC, Loscalzo J (eds): Cecil Essentials of Medicine, ed 6. Philadelphia, Saunders, 2004
10. Beckerman J, Wang P, Hlatky M: Cardiovascular screening of athletes. Clin J Sport Med 2004;14(3):127-133
11. 26th Bethesda Conference: recommendations for determining eligibility for competition in athletes with cardiovascular abnormalities. January 6-7, 1994. Med Sci Sports Exerc 1994;26(10 suppl):S223-283 [published erratum in Med Sci Sports Exerc 1994;26(12):following table of contents]
12. Maron BJ, Chaitman BR, Ackerman MJ, et al: Recommendations for physical activity and recreational sports participation for young patients with genetic cardiovascular diseases, AHA Scientific Statement. Circulation 2004;109(22):2807-2816
13. American Academy of Family Physicians, American Academy of Pediatrics, American Medical Society for Sports Medicine, American Orthopaedic Society for Sports Medicine, American Osteopathic Academy of Sports Medicine: Preparticipation Physical Evaluation, ed 2. Minneapolis, New York City, McGraw-Hill Inc, 1997, p 20
14. Carek PJ, Mainous A III: The preparticipation physical examination for athletics: a systematic review of current recommendations. BMJ USA 2003;2:661-664
15. Bender TW III: Cutaneous manifestations of disease in athletes. Skinmed 2003;2(1):34-40
16. Brooks C, Kujawska A, Patel D: Cutaneous allergic reactions induced by sporting activities. Sports Med 2003;33(9): 699-708
17. Metelitsa A, Marankin B, Lin AN: Diagnosis of sports-related dermatoses. Int J Dermatol 2004;43(2):113-119
18. Gomez JE, Landry GL, Bernhardt DT: Critical evaluation of the 2-minute orthopedic screening examination. Am J Dis Child 1993;147(10):1109-1113
19. Rifat SF, Ruffin MT, Gorenflo DW: Disqualifying criteria in a preparticipation sports evaluation. J Fam Pract 1995;41(1):42-50

20. Smith J, Laskowski ER: The preparticipation physical examination: Mayo Clinic experience with 2,739 examinations. Mayo Clin Proc 1998;73(5):419-429
21. De Paepe A, Devereux RB, Dietz HC, et al: Revised diagnostic criteria for the Marfan syndrome. Am J Med Genet 1996; 62(4):417-426
22. Lombardo JA, Robinson JB, Smith DM, et al: Preparticipation Physical Evaluation, ed 1. Kansas City, MO, American Academy of Family Physicians, American Academy of Pediatrics, American Medical Society for Sports Medicine, American Orthopaedic Society for Sports Medicine, American Osteopathic Academy of Sports Medicine, 1992
23. Smith DM: Preparticipation physical evaluations: development of uniform guidelines. Sports Med 1994;18(5):293-300
24. Kelly BT, Kadrmas WR, Speer KP: The manual muscle examination for rotator cuff strength: an electromyographic investigation. Am J Sports Med 1996;24(5):581-588
25. Speer KP, Hannafin JA, Altchek DW, et al: An evaluation of the shoulder relocation test. Am J Sports Med 1994;22(2):177-183
26. Katz K, Rosenthal A, Yosipovitch Z: Normal ranges of popliteal angle in children. J Pediatr Orthop 1992;12(2):229-231

27. Gajdosik R, Lusin G: Hamstring muscle tightness: Reliability of an active knee-extension test. Phys Ther 1983;63(7):1085-1090
28. Kim SJ, Kim HK: Reliability of the anterior drawer test, the pivot shift test, and the Lachman test. Clin Orthop 1995; Aug (317):237-242
29. Kibler WB, Chandler TJ, Uhl T, et al: A musculoskeletal approach to the preparticipation physical examination: preventing injury and improving performance. Am J Sports Med 1989;17(4):525-531
30. Kibler WB, Chandler TJ: Sport specific screening and testing, in Renstrom P (ed): Sports Injuries: Basic Principles of Prevention and Care: Olympic Encyclopedia of Sports Medicine, vol 4. Oxford, Boston, Blackwell Sccientific Pubs, 1993
31. Amir D, Frankl U, Pogrund H: Pulled elbow and hypermobility of joints. Clin Orthop 1990;Aug(257):94-99
32. Decoster LC, Vailas JC, Lindsay RH, et al: Prevalence and features of joint hypermobility among adolescent athletes. Arch Pediatr Adolesc Med 1997;151(10):989-992
33. Didia BC, Dapper DV, Boboye SB: Joint hypermobility syndrome among undergraduate students. East Afr Med J 2002;79(2):80-81

Chapter 7

DETERMINING CLEARANCE

etermining clearance is an important and sometimes difficult decision. Studies of the PPE show that 3.1% to 13.9% of athletes require further evaluation before a final clearance status can be determined.[1-11]

The initial clearance status for an athlete can be divided into 4 categories:

◆ Cleared without restriction;

◆ Cleared, with recommendations for further evaluation or treatment (eg, "recheck blood pressure in 1 month");

◆ Not cleared—clearance status to be reconsidered after completion of further evaluation, treatment, or rehabilitation; and

◆ Not cleared for certain types of sports or for all sports.

Forms for recording clearance status are available on page 95.

◤ CLEARANCE CONSIDERATIONS

It must be reemphasized that the PPE is not intended to discourage or prevent participation in competitive sports. All athletes deserve a diligent and thorough assessment of any issues that could lead to denial of participation. Should such an evaluation result in restriction from participation in the sport of choice, the physician must consider alternative forms of participation. The decision to restrict participation may prevent an individual from reaping the many health benefits of regular physical exercise and may cause significant psychological consequences. One study[12] emphasized the importance of participation by pointing out that adolescents rank failure to make a team worse than the death of a close friend, failure to pass a grade in school, and separation of parents.

When an abnormality or condition is found that may limit an athlete's participation or predispose him or her to further injury, the physician must consider the following questions:

◆ Does the problem place the athlete at increased risk for injury or illness?

◆ Is another participant at risk for injury or illness because of the problem?

◆ Can the athlete safely participate with treatment (such as medication, rehabilitation, bracing, or padding)?

◆ Can limited participation be allowed while treatment is being completed?

◆ If clearance is denied only for certain sports or sport categories, in what activities can the athlete safely participate?

When a potentially disqualifying issue is identified during the PPE, clearance for a particular sport should be considered based on a review of the pertinent current literature. Examples include guidelines established by the AAP Committee on Sports Medicine and Fitness (tables 21, 22, and 23) and the 26th Bethesda Conference guidelines on cardiovascular abnormalities.[13,14] These recommendations classify sports according to the degree of contact and the level of dynamic and static stress.

Contact categories (see table 21) are based on the potential for injury from collision. High-impact contact-collision sports, such as football and ice hockey, have a higher risk of serious injury than do noncontact sports, such as golf.

Distinctions based on strenuousness (see table 22) are particularly relevant for athletes with cardiovascular or pulmonary disease. Static exercise causes a pressure load, whereas dynamic exercise causes a volume load on the left ventricle.[15]

In all cases, the physician's judgment is essential in applying these recommendations to a specific patient.

It is the opinion of the author societies that clearance status is best determined when the PPE is conducted using the single–physician examiner model. Should the PPE be performed with multiple examiners, clearance should be determined by a physician who has reviewed the entire history and physical exam. In any PPE format, clearance is best determined by a physician who is familiar with the demands of the activities, the limitations that result from various problems, and the current medical literature on what affects safe participation. The physician may also decide on follow-up and further workup for a specific problem found during the PPE, whether or not it affects participation. The physician determining clearance should refer to the relevant recommendations

Table 21 — Classification of Sports by Contact

Contact or Collision	Limited Contact	Noncontact
Basketball	Baseball	Archery
Boxing*	Bicycling	Badminton
Diving	Cheerleading	Body building
Field hockey	Canoeing or kayaking	Bowling
Football, tackle	(white water)	Canoeing or kayaking
Ice hockey†	Fencing	(flat water)
Lacrosse	Field events	Crew or rowing
Martial arts	High jump	Curling
Rodeo	Pole vault	Dancing§
Rugby	Floor hockey	Ballet
Ski jumping	Football, flag	Modern
Soccer	Gymnastics	Jazz
Team handball	Handball	Field events
Water polo	Horseback riding	Discus
Wrestling	Racquetball	Javelin
	Skating	Shot put
	Ice	Golf
	In-line	Orienteering‖
	Roller	Power lifting
	Skiing	Race walking
	Cross-country	Riflery
	Downhill	Rope jumping
	Water	Running
	Skateboarding	Sailing
	Snowboarding‡	Scuba diving
	Softball	Swimming
	Squash	Table tennis
	Ultimate frisbee	Tennis
	Volleyball	Track
	Windsurfing or surfing	Weight lifting

*Participation not recommended by the AAP.
†The AAP recommends limiting the amount of body checking allowed for hockey players 15 years and younger to reduce injuries.
‡Snowboarding has been added since previous statement was published.
§Dancing has been further classified into ballet, modern, and jazz since the previous monograph was published.
‖A race in which competitors use a map and compass to find their way through unfamiliar territory.

Reprinted with permission from: American Academy of Pediatrics Committee on Sports Medicine and Fitness: Medical conditions affecting sports participation. Pediatrics 2001;107(5):1205-1209.

needed to establish the clearance status of the athlete or seek appropriate consultation as needed.

No matter which type of PPE format is used, it is extremely important to ensure complete understanding by the athletes and parent(s) of any restrictions, necessary workup and treatment, and any alternative activities in which the athlete may participate. While athletic trainers, coaches, and school administrators can be informed of the general participation status of the athlete, confidentiality must be maintained. The dissemination of any medical information must be done in accordance with federal laws concerning privacy of medical records (see "Administrative and Legal Concerns," chapter 4, page 11).

Using a clearance form separate from the history and physical examination form, such as that on page 95, is suggested to provide the parents and school with a copy of clearance decisions and follow-up recommendations while protecting the confidentiality of athletes' history and physical findings. Alternatively,

Table 22 — Classification of Sports by Strenuousness

High-to-Moderate Intensity

High-to-Moderate Dynamic and Static Demands	High-to-Moderate Dynamic and Low Static Demands	High-to-Moderate Static and Low Dynamic Demands
Boxing*	Badminton	Archery
Crew or rowing	Baseball	Auto racing
Cross-country skiing	Basketball	Diving
Cycling	Field hockey	Horseback riding (jumping)
Downhill skiing	Lacrosse	Field events (throwing)
Fencing	Orienteering	Gymnastics
Football	Race walking	Karate or judo
Ice hockey	Racquetball	Motorcycling
Rugby	Soccer	Rodeo
Running (sprint)	Squash	Sailing
Speed skating	Swimming	Ski jumping
Water polo	Table tennis	Waterskiing
Wrestling	Tennis	Weight lifting
	Volleyball	

Low Intensity

Low Dynamic and Low Static Demands
Bowling
Cricket
Curling
Golf
Riflery

*Participation not recommended by the AAP.

Reprinted with permission from: American Academy of Pediatrics Committee on Sports Medicine and Fitness: Medical conditions affecting sports participation. Pediatrics 2001;107(5):1205-1209.

this form may be used just for athletes who are not fully cleared.

In some cases, the school or organization may have a designated team physician who was not part of the PPE process. In such situations, it may be appropriate for the physician who performed the PPE to seek permission from the student-athlete and parent(s) to communicate to the team physician any ongoing problems that could affect safe participation.

Occasionally, an athlete will wish to participate despite medical recommendations to the contrary. In such cases, it is critical that the athlete, parent(s) or guardian(s), coach, and school or program administrators all understand the degree of risk in participation and the potential long-term consequences of participation. (See page 11 for a discussion of participation rights and exculpatory waivers.)

◣ MEDICATION AND SUPPLEMENT USE

During the PPE, physicians may often be asked questions regarding the use of medications and supplements, or they may identify athletes who have been using substances for performance enhancement. Such individuals should be counseled regarding the safety and effectiveness of such agents, as well as issues related to drug testing.

Competitors need to be aware of the names and dosages of any drugs and supplements they are taking, as well as the policies that affect them. Recent studies show that supplements may contain substances that are not listed on the label that are banned by various sports organizations, and that the amount of the substances that are listed may vary considerably.[16] Athletes who are subject to drug testing by a sport organization

Table 23 — Medical Conditions and Sports Participation*

Condition	May Participate
Atlantoaxial instability (instability of the joint between cervical vertebrae 1 and 2) Explanation: Athlete needs evaluation to assess risk of spinal cord injury during sports participation.	**Qualified yes**
Bleeding disorder† Explanation: Athlete needs evaluation.	**Qualified yes**
Cardiovascular disease	
Carditis (inflammation of the heart) Explanation: Carditis may result in sudden death with exertion.	**No**
Hypertension (high blood pressure) Explanation: Those with significant essential (unexplained) hypertension should avoid weight and power lifting, body building, and strength training. Those with secondary hypertension (hypertension caused by a previously identified disease) or severe essential hypertension need evaluation. The National High Blood Pressure Education Working group defined significant and severe hypertension (see tables 16 and 17, page 47).	**Qualified yes**
Congenital heart disease (structural heart defects present at birth) Explanation: Those with mild forms may participate fully; those with moderate or severe forms or who have undergone surgery need evaluation. The 26th Bethesda Conference defined mild, moderate, and severe disease for common cardiac lesions.	**Qualified yes**
Dysrhythmia (irregular heart rhythm) Explanation: Those with symptoms (chest pain, syncope, dizziness, shortness of breath, or other symptoms of possible dysrhythmia) or evidence of mitral regurgitation (leaking) on physical examination need evaluation. All others may participate fully.	**Qualified yes**
Heart murmur Explanation: If the murmur is innocent (does not indicate heart disease), full participation is permitted. Otherwise, the athlete needs evaluation (see "Congenital heart disease," above, and mitral valve prolapse discussion in the text).	**Qualified yes**
Cerebral palsy† Explanation: Athlete needs evaluation.	**Qualified yes**
Diabetes mellitus Explanation: All sports can be played with proper attention to diet, blood glucose concentration, hydration, and insulin therapy. Blood glucose concentration should be monitored every 30 minutes during continuous exercise and 15 minutes after completion of exercise.	**Yes**
Diarrhea Explanation: Unless disease is mild, no participation is permitted, because diarrhea may increase the risk of dehydration and heat illness. See "Fever," below.	**Qualified no**
Eating disorders	
Anorexia nervosa, bulimia nervosa Explanation: Patients with these disorders need medical and psychiatric assessment before participation.	**Qualified yes**
Eyes	
Functionally 1-eyed athlete, loss of an eye, detached retina, previous eye surgery, or serious eye injury Explanation: A functionally 1-eyed athlete has a best-corrected visual acuity of less than 20/40 in the eye with worse acuity. These athletes would suffer significant disability if the better eye were seriously injured, as would those with loss of an eye. Some athletes who previously have undergone eye surgery or had a serious eye injury may have an increased risk of injury because of weakened eye tissue. Availability of eye guards approved by the American Society for Testing and Materials and other protective equipment may allow participation in most sports, but this must be judged on an individual basis (see table 25 on page 71).	**Qualified yes**
Fever Explanation: Fever can increase cardiopulmonary effort, reduce maximum exercise capacity, make heat illness more likely, and increase orthostatic hypertension during exercise. Fever may rarely accompany myocarditis or other infections that may make exercise dangerous.	**No**
Heat illness, history of Explanation: Because of the increased likelihood of recurrence, the athlete needs individual assessment to determine the presence of predisposing conditions and to arrange a prevention strategy.	**Qualified yes**
Hepatitis Explanation: Because of the apparent minimal risk to others, all sports may be played that the athlete's state of health allows. In all athletes, skin lesions should be covered properly, and athletic personnel should use universal precautions when handling blood or body fluids with visible blood.	**Yes**
Human immunodeficiency virus (HIV) infection Explanation: Because of the apparent minimal risk to others, all sports may be played that the athlete's state of health allows. In all athletes, skin lesions should be covered properly, and athletic personnel should use universal precautions when handling blood or body fluids with visible blood.	**Yes**

Condition	May Participate
Kidney, absence of one Explanation: Athlete needs individual assessment for contact, collision, and limited-contact sports.	**Qualified yes**
Liver, enlarged Explanation: If the liver is acutely enlarged, participation should be avoided because of risk of rupture. If the liver is chronically enlarged, individual assessment is needed before collision, contact, or limited-contact sports are played.	**Qualified yes**
Malignant neoplasm† Explanation: Athlete needs individual assessment.	**Qualified yes**
Musculoskeletal disorders Explanation: Athlete needs individual assessment.	**Qualified yes**
Neurologic disorders **History of serious head or spine trauma, severe or repeated concussions, or craniotomy** Explanation: Athlete needs individual assessment for collision, contact, or limited-contact sports and also for noncontact sports if deficits in judgment or cognition are present. Research supports a conservative approach to management of concussion.	**Qualified yes**
Seizure disorder, well-controlled Explanation: Risk of seizure during participation is minimal.	**Yes**
Seizure disorder, poorly controlled Explanation: Athlete needs individual assessment for collision, contact, or limited-contact sports. The following noncontact sports should be avoided: archery, riflery, swimming, weight or power lifting, strength training, or sports involving heights. In these sports, occurrence of a seizure may pose a risk to self or others.	**Qualified yes**
Obesity Explanation: Because of the risk of heat illness, obese persons need careful acclimatization and hydration.	**Qualified yes**
Organ transplant recipient† Explanation: Athlete needs individual assessment.	**Qualified yes**
Ovary, absence of one Explanation: Risk of severe injury to the remaining ovary is minimal.	**Yes**
Respiratory conditions **Pulmonary compromise, including cystic fibrosis** Explanation: Athlete needs individual assessment, but generally, all sports may be played if oxygenation remains satisfactory during a graded exercise test. Patients with cystic fibrosis need acclimatization and good hydration to reduce the risk of heat illness.	**Qualified yes**
Asthma Explanation: With proper medication and education, only athletes with the most severe asthma will need to modify their participation.	**Yes**
Acute upper respiratory infection Explanation: Upper respiratory obstruction may affect pulmonary function. Athlete needs individual assessment for all but mild disease. See "Fever," on previous page.	**Qualified yes**
Sickle cell disease Explanation: Athlete needs individual assessment. In general, if status of the illness permits, all but high exertion, collision, and contact sports may be played. Overheating, dehydration, and chilling must be avoided.	**Qualified yes**
Sickle cell trait Explanation: It is unlikely that persons with sickle cell trait have an increased risk of sudden death or other medical problems during athletic participation, except under the most extreme conditions of heat, humidity, and, possibly, increased altitude. These persons, like all athletes, should be carefully conditioned, acclimatized, and hydrated to reduce any possible risk.	**Yes**
Skin disorders (boils, herpes simplex, impetigo, scabies, molluscum contagiosum) Explanation: While the patient is contagious, participation in gymnastics with mats; martial arts; wrestling; or other collision, contact, or limited-contact sports is not allowed.	**Qualified yes**
Spleen, enlarged Explanation: A patient with an acutely enlarged spleen should avoid all sports because of risk of rupture. A patient with a chronically enlarged spleen needs individual assessment before playing collision, contact, or limited-contact sports.	**Qualified yes**
Testicle, undescended or absence of one Explanation: Certain sports may require a protective cup.	**Yes**

*This table is designed for use by medical and nonmedical personnel. "Needs evaluation" means that a physician with appropriate knowledge and experience should assess the safety of a given sport for an athlete with the listed medical condition. Unless otherwise noted, this is because of variability of the severity of the disease, the risk of injury for the specific sports listed in table 21 (page 62), or both.
†Not discussed in the text of the monograph.

Reprinted with permission from: American Academy of Pediatrics Committee on Sports Medicine and Fitness: Medical conditions affecting sports participation. Pediatrics 2001;107(5):1205-1209.

are responsible for the content of any substance they ingest. A positive test that results from using a product without knowing its contents, or a product whose contents are inaccurately labeled, may nonetheless result in sanctions. With respect to drug testing, athletes should therefore be advised that those who use such products do so at their own risk.

Sports medicine physicians should be familiar with the drug testing guidelines relevant to their institution. In addition, athletes may be competing for multiple organizations with varying drug-testing regulations. Physicians should therefore be cognizant of this when counseling athletes and when prescribing medications. *Any physician prescribing medication to an athlete subject to drug testing should ensure that it is not a banned substance.* If a medication needed to treat a condition is on the banned list and no alternative is available, the sport organization should be contacted to determine if approval for use of the medication can be obtained. Up-to-date information regarding drug testing and banned substances may be obtained from the following sources:

◆ *NCAA Sports Medicine Handbook and Drug Testing Program Book:* Can be ordered via the Web (www.ncaa.org) or by phone (888-388-9748); the Web site provides printable files of these publications, including the banned drug list.

◆ USADA: Provides a drug reference hotline: 1-800-233-0393; additional information, including banned substance lists and printable reference material, can be obtained at www.usantidoping.org.

ACUTE ILLNESS

On occasion, the physician performing the PPE may encounter an athlete experiencing an acute illness. Because the PPE is performed in advance of the sports season, denial of participation because of an acute illness does not generally occur. However, the ability of the athlete to safely participate in training and conditioning may be affected until the illness has resolved.

When such a situation occurs, clearance should be based on individual assessment. Factors to consider include the risk of the illness worsening as a result of participation and the potential for spreading the disease to others. The author societies recommend restriction of participation for athletes with a febrile illness and those with ongoing fluid losses due to gas-trointestinal illnesses. Limiting activity in such patients is important in preventing complications such as dehydration, thermoregulatory problems, and viral myocarditis—although the latter is rare.

BLOODBORNE PATHOGENS: HIV AND HEPATITIS

The bloodborne pathogens of greatest concern in sports are human immunodeficiency virus (HIV) and the hepatitis B and C viruses (HBV and HCV). All can be transmitted through parenteral exposure to blood and blood products, contamination of open wounds or mucous membranes with infected blood, sexual contact, and perinatal spread from an infected mother to her baby. Body piercing and tattoos may also present some risk of contracting HIV, HCV, and HBV. Further, the sharing of needles during the use of injectable anabolic steroids has been reported to result in HIV transmission and may increase the risk of contracting HBV and HCV.[17,18]

Although HIV is present in tears, sweat, urine, sputum, vomitus, saliva, and respiratory droplets, only blood is recognized as a threat in the athletic setting. HIV transmission during sports has not been documented. One published report[19] described a suspected case in an Italian soccer player. However, this report was poorly documented and has not been accepted as a transmission related to sport. Transmission of HIV has never been shown to occur in the NFL. The *risk of transmission* has been estimated to be less than 1 occurrence per 85 million games.[20]

Although HBV is more concentrated in blood and more easily transmitted than HIV among healthcare workers, HBV transmission in sports is rare.[21] There have been 2 reports of HBV transmission during sports.[22,23] In the United States, the practice of routine HBV immunization further reduces the risk of transmission.

HCV was recognized as a cause of non-A, non-B hepatitis in 1988.[24] The risk of transmission of HCV to healthcare workers exposed to infected blood is intermediate to HIV and HBV.[21,24] Transmission of HCV via exposure during sports participation has not been documented.

Thus, the risk of transmitting HIV, HBV, and HCV in sports is not zero, but, because it is so uncommon, it has not been quantifiable.[25] Sports that involve close body contact for sustained periods (such as wrestling) are considered to present a relatively higher risk of transmission. Nonetheless, the risk is considered minimal.[21,25,26]

Since HIV, HBV, and HCV appear to present minimal risk to others, the NCAA, AAP, AMSSM, and American Academy of Sports Medicine do not view the presence of such infections alone as a reason for exclusion from participation.[21,25,26] Asymptomatic individuals may participate in sports under the guidance and ongoing monitoring of a knowledgeable physician. Clinical signs and symptoms should be evaluated in relation to the demands of the sport. The type of athletic activity, the health risks of participation, intensity of training, and risk of transmission to others all need to be considered. Changes in the affected athlete's health status mandate reevaluation of the participation level. Finally, confidentiality of the health status of the individual must be maintained.

◣ CARDIOVASCULAR ABNORMALITIES

Clearance guidelines for cardiovascular conditions in young athletes have been established by considering which conditions may be exacerbated by physical activity and which predispose an athlete to sudden cardiac death. The guidelines established by the 26th Bethesda Conference[14] cover the major cardiac abnormalities seen in athletes, including hypertension, arrhythmias, congenital heart disease, acquired valvular disease, ischemic heart disease, and the cardiomyopathies. It is recommended that any physician who is determining clearance for an athlete with a cardiovascular condition consult this reference, as well as more recent recommendations cited below. If any doubts remain about the cardiovascular condition after thorough evaluation by the athlete's personal physician, the athlete should not be cleared until evaluation by a cardiologist has been completed. Summaries for selected common cardiac conditions follow.

Hypertension. Elevated blood pressure is one of the most common abnormalities found during the PPE.[2,4,10,11] Care should be taken to ensure accurate blood pressure measurement according to the Seventh Report of the Joint National Committee on Prevention, Detection, Evaluation, and Treatment of High Blood Pressure (JNC 7).[27] In particular, appropriately sized blood pressure cuffs should be available during screening to obtain accurate readings.

Previous recommendations concerning the participation status of athletes with hypertension were based on the 26th Bethesda Conference report.[14] The following recommendations reflect an update that takes into consideration the most recent blood pressure classification guidelines for children and adults (see tables 16 and 17 on page 47).[27,28]

Athletes 18 years old and older who are identified during the PPE as having a blood pressure reading classified as prehypertension or stage 1 hypertension according to the JNC 7, and who have no evidence of target organ damage, may compete in all categories of sports. Such individuals should be under the care of a physician and receive regular monitoring of their blood pressure.

Those who are found to have stage 2 hypertension (systolic blood pressure ≥ 160 mm Hg or diastolic blood pressure ≥ 100 mm Hg), or who have findings of end-organ damage, should not be allowed to participate in any competitive sport until their blood pressure is further evaluated and treated, at which time eligibility for participation can be reevaluated. Cardiovascular conditioning activities may be considered in such cases on an individual basis.

For those younger than 18, normative blood pressures have been established based on age, gender, and height.[28] Children and adolescents with a blood pressure measurement greater than the 99th percentile for age, gender, and height—or who have evidence of end-organ damage—are managed similar to adults with stage 2 hypertension as described above. Those with a blood pressure measurement above the 90th percentile but less than the 99th percentile, and who do not have findings of target-organ damage, may participate while undergoing additional assessment and treatment.

Therefore, unless: (1) hypertension first noted at the PPE is at the stage 2 level in an adult or greater than the 99th percentile for children, (2) there is a concern that end-organ damage exists, or (3) a secondary cause of hypertension is suspected, the athlete may be cleared for competition while undergoing further evaluation.

Benign functional murmurs. These are commonly found during the PPE but do not preclude participation in sports (see also pages 21 and 48).

Mitral valve prolapse should not result in restriction

from participation in high-intensity competitive sports unless accompanied by 1 of the following: (1) history of syncope due to arrhythmia, (2) family history of sudden death attributed to mitral valve prolapse, (3) prior embolic event, (4) arrhythmia (eg, supraventricular arrhythmias) worsened by exercise, or (5) moderate-to-marked mitral regurgitation. If any of these criteria apply, participation in low-intensity sports may be considered on an individual basis.

Hypertrophic cardiomyopathy. Athletes with an unequivocal diagnosis of HCM—the most common cause of sudden death in young athletes in the United States[29]—should not be allowed to participate in competitive sports, with the possible exception of low-intensity sports as defined by the 26th Bethesda conference. Though some nationally known athletes have been allowed to engage in high-dynamic sports, risk stratification for athletes with HCM is especially difficult because of the extreme conditions that can occur with high-intensity training and competition. In addition, recent data suggest that removal of athletes with HCM from competitive sports may reduce the risk for sudden cardiac death.[30]

Advances in the treatment of HCM have included the use of implantable cardioverter defibrillators (ICDs) to prevent death. ICD placement is currently recommended for secondary prevention of sudden cardiac death in those with a prior cardiac arrest or sustained, spontaneous ventricular tachycardia.[31] ICD use is also considered in the primary prevention of sudden cardiac death for those deemed at high risk because of multiple clinical risk factors or a single major risk factor (eg, family history of sudden death from HCM). However, there is no published literature regarding the use of ICDs for primary prevention in HCM patients considered at low risk who are then exposed to the rigors of competitive sports. The American College of Cardiology/European Society of Cardiology clinical expert consensus document on hypertrophic cardiomyopathy reviewed these recent developments in HCM and supports the recommendation that individuals with HCM should avoid exposure to most competitive sports.[31]

Arrhythmias. Although a detailed discussion of arrhythmias is beyond the scope of this monograph, recommendations for clearance of athletes are covered in the 26th Bethesda Conference guidelines and the more recent Expert Consensus Conference on Arrhyth-

mias in the Athlete of the North American Society of Pacing and Electrophysiology.[14,32]

DERMATOLOGIC DISORDERS

The presence of any open wound or infectious skin condition that cannot be protected in order to prevent exposure to other athletes warrants exclusion from competition.[33] Examples include herpes simplex, scabies, louse infestation, molluscum contagiosum, tinea corporis, impetigo, and furuncles or carbuncles. In particular, herpes gladiatorum and tinea corporis gladiatorum are notoriously problematic.

Denying clearance is especially important in sports in which close physical contact occurs, such as wrestling, rugby, and martial arts, and in sports in which equipment such as baseball helmets is shared. Recent studies suggest that prompt identification and treatment of infected athletes is essential to prevent the spread of the infection to teammates and competitors.[34] Participation may be resumed when the condition has been adequately treated and is no longer contagious. For athletes with recurrent herpes gladiatorum, nucleoside analogues (eg, acyclovir, famciclovir, or valacyclovir) are effective in preventing recurrence and are therefore recommended.[35]

Outbreaks of community-associated methicillin-resistant *Staphylococcus aureus* (CA-MRSA) skin infections have recently been described among competitive athletes.[36,37] Since any open skin lesion is a potential site for the development of CA-MRSA, skin wounds identified during the PPE (or at any time) should be promptly treated and covered. Athletes should be reminded to avoid sharing of personal items, including towels and razors. Athletes with CA-MRSA should be treated with appropriate antibiotics. They may return to play when the infection is clinically controlled as determined by the treating physician and the wound is able to be adequately covered.

The specific requirements for return to participation for wrestlers with skin infections can be obtained from the NFHS and the NCAA.[38,39]

DIABETES MELLITUS

It is important that those with a history of type 1 or type 2 diabetes mellitus be carefully screened for signs of complications that could affect participation status, including: cardiovascular disease (hypertension and coronary artery disease), peripheral vascular disease, retinopathy, nephropathy, neuropathy (peripheral and autonomic), and gastrointestinal problems (gastroparesis).[40-42]

For patients with coronary artery disease or peripheral vascular disease, an appropriate level of activity should be determined by the treating primary physician or specialist. In patients with retinopathy, strenuous exercise can cause retinal detachment or vitreal hemorrhage. The American Diabetes Association recommends that activities that significantly elevate blood pressure, such as weight lifting, be avoided in those with moderate or severe nonproliferative retinopathy.[42] These activities, and also high-impact activities (eg, jogging), should also be avoided by those with proliferative retinopathy.

There are little data on how strenuous exercise affects diabetic nephropathy, though the presence of this complication may limit exercise capacity. Highly strenuous activities should most likely be restricted, though each case should be managed on an individual basis.[42]

Those with peripheral neuropathy can injure their feet during exercise. Because of this, it is recommended that their activities be limited to those that do not cause repetitive impact to the feet (eg, bicycling and swimming).[42]

Patients with autonomic neuropathy must be screened for coronary artery disease. They can have difficulty exercising in hot or cold environments due to thermoregulatory dysfunction. Postural hypotension may also occur. The activity level of these individuals may therefore be significantly limited. The examining physician may indicate which activities are acceptable on a case-by-case basis.

Diabetic gastroparesis can affect fluid and electrolyte absorption and thus may limit safe participation in strenuous activities, prolonged activities, or activities performed in warm environments.

Because of the risk of hypoglycemia during exercise, sports such as rock climbing, skydiving, and scuba diving are considered high risk for diabetic individuals.[43] Solo endurance activities (eg, ultramarathons, cycling, open-water swimming) may make it difficult to have proper support available for diabetic athletes to ensure safe participation. And motor sports present a potential risk to other competitors. Although the use of insulin pumps may reduce the frequency of hypo-

glycemia in those with type 1 diabetes and are now being used by athletes, such activities remain high risk.[44]

Those with diabetes who are free of complications and who are in good blood glucose control should not be restricted from participation in sports that do not present a high risk. Furthermore, the increasing use of intensive insulin therapy and insulin pumps has given athletes who have diabetes greater ability in adjusting insulin dosing to suit their activities. Although a complete discussion of the management of diabetes in athletes is beyond the scope of this document, the American Diabetes Association provides the following general guidelines for regulating blood glucose in athletes with type 1 diabetes[42]:

1. Metabolic control before exercise.

◆ Avoid exercise if fasting glucose levels are greater than 250 mg/dL and ketosis is present or if glucose levels are greater than 300 mg/dL, irrespective of whether ketosis is present.

◆ Ingest added carbohydrate if glucose levels are less than 100 mg/dL.

2. Blood glucose monitoring before and after exercise.

◆ Identify when changes in insulin or food intake are necessary.

◆ Learn the glycemic response to different exercise conditions.

3. Food intake.

◆ Consume added carbohydrate as needed to avoid hypoglycemia.

◆ Carbohydrate-based foods should be readily available during and after exercise.

In addition, the athlete with diabetes should be well instructed on maintaining adequate hydration, using proper footwear, and monitoring the feet for skin trauma. All these patients should wear a diabetes identification bracelet or shoe tag.

◤ DISORDERED EATING AND THE FEMALE ATHLETE TRIAD

When disordered eating alone or the female athlete triad (interrelated disordered eating, amenorrhea, and osteopenia or osteoporosis) is suspected, evaluation and treatment, using a multidisciplinary approach, is warranted.[45] In addition, recent research has emphasized the role of inadequate energy availability in the development of oligomenorrhea or amenorrhea and osteopenia or osteoporosis in athletes.[46-48] That is, individuals who do not display disordered eating behavior of psychological origin may develop oligomenorrhea or amenorrhea or have lower bone mineral density simply due to inadequate caloric intake. Athletes may be reluctant to undergo treatment, but their cooperation is imperative. It must be stressed to coaches and athletes that inadequate caloric intake or disordered eating behaviors may impair athletic performance and predispose the athlete to injury, particularly stress fractures.[48]

Athletic participation should be restricted when there is evidence of compromised performance or when disordered eating or the female athlete triad has threatened the athlete's health in such a way that continued participation could cause injury or deterioration of the athlete's health status.

◣ EYE DISORDERS AND ABNORMAL VISION

The potential for loss of vision because of injury is always a concern in sports. Although it is difficult to quantify the relative risk of eye injury for a specific sport, some sports such as basketball, baseball, softball, ice hockey, field hockey, and lacrosse are classified as high risk because of the number of eye injuries reported and the potential for eye impact sufficient to cause injury.[49] Table 24 provides the eye injury risk classification for a variety of sports.

Because protective devices exist that can significantly reduce the risk of eye injury, it is important that all athletes and their parent(s) are made aware of the types of eye protection available and the risks of the particular sport. It is essential to consider eye protection for athletes whose vision is already impaired in 1 eye. A visual acuity of 20/40 or better in at least 1 eye is considered to provide good vision. An individual is deemed functionally 1-eyed if the loss of the better eye would result in a significant change in lifestyle. Consequently, athletes with best corrected vision in 1 eye of less than 20/40 should be considered functionally 1-eyed.[50]

Sports in which eye protection cannot be effectively worn are contraindicated for functionally 1-eyed athletes. Athletes who are functionally 1-eyed and who participate in sports that carry a high risk of eye injury may be individually evaluated and allowed to participate if they wear appropriate protective eyewear (table 25).

The athlete, his or her parent(s) or guardian(s), the coach, and school administrators, if necessary, must

Table 24	**Categories of Sports-Related Eye-Injury Risk to the Unprotected Player**

High Risk

Small, fast projectiles
Air rifle
BB gun
Paintball

Hard projectiles, "sticks," close contact
Baseball/softball
Basketball
Cricket
Fencing
Hockey (field and ice)
Lacrosse (men's and women's)
Racquetball
Squash

Intentional injury
Boxing
Full-contact martial arts

Moderate Risk

Badminton
Fishing
Football
Golf
Soccer
Tennis
Volleyball
Water polo

Low Risk

Bicycling
Diving
Noncontact martial arts
Skiing (snow and water)
Swimming
Wrestling

Eye Safe

Gymnastics
Track and field*

*Javelin and discus have a small but definite potential for injury. However, good field supervision can reduce the extremely low risk of injury to nearly negligible.

Adapted with permission from: Vinger PF: A practical guide for sports eye protection. Phys Sportmed 2000; 28(6):49-69. Available at: http://www.physsportsmed.com/issues/2000/06_00/vinger.htm.

understand: (1) the serious long-term consequences if injury to the better eye were to occur, (2) the level of protection available for the better eye, and (3) the degree of

| Table 25 | Recommended Eye Protectors for Selected Sports |

Sport	Minimal Eye Protector	Comment
Baseball/softball (youth batter and base runner)	ASTM standard F910	Face guard attached to helmet
Baseball/softball (fielder)	ASTM standard F803 for baseball	ASTM specifies age ranges
Basketball	ASTM standard F803 for basketball	ASTM specifies age ranges
Bicycling	Helmet plus street wear/fashion eyewear	
Boxing	None available; not permitted in the sport	Contraindicated for functionally 1-eyed athletes
Fencing	Protector with neck bib	
Field hockey (men's and women's)	ASTM standard F803 for women's lacrosse (goalie: full face mask)	Protectors that pass for women's lacrosse also pass for field hockey
Football	Polycarbonate eye shield attached to helmet-mounted wire face mask	
Full-contact martial arts	None available; not permitted in the sport	Contraindicated for functionally 1-eyed athletes
Ice hockey	ASTM standard F513 face mask on helmet (goaltenders: ASTM standard F1587)	HECC- OR CSA-certified full-face shield
Lacrosse (men's)	Face mask attached to lacrosse helmet	
Lacrosse (women's)	ASTM standard F803 for women's lacrosse	Should have option to wear helmet
Paintball	ASTM standard F1776 for paintball	
Racket sports (badminton, tennis, paddle tennis, handball, squash, and racquetball)	ASTM standard F803 for selected sport	
Soccer	ASTM standard F803 for selected sport	
Street hockey	ASTM standard F513 face mask on helmet	Must be HECC or CSA certified
Track and field	Street wear with polycarbonate lenses/fashion eyewear*	
Water polo/swimming	Swim goggles with polycarbonate lenses	
Wrestling	No standard available	Custom protective eyewear can be made

*Eyewear that passes ASTM standard F803 is safer than street wear eyewear for all sports activities with impact potential.
ASTM = American Society for Testing and Materials; HECC = Hockey Equipment Certification Council; CSA = Canadian Standards Association
Adapted with permission from: Vinger PF: A practical guide for sports eye protection. Phys Sportmed 2000;28(6):49-69.
Available at: http://www.physsportsmed.com/issues/2000/06_00/vinger.htm.

risk of injury—with and without protection—to the better eye. Treatments for injuries that can typically occur in the desired activity should also be discussed.

If, after this discussion, the functionally 1-eyed athlete still wishes to participate in a given sport, he or she must wear appropriate protective eyewear during participation (see also pages 11 and 61).

Athletes with eye conditions, including a high degree of myopia, surgical aphakia, retinal detachment, and a history of eye surgery, injury, or infection, may be at increased risk for eye injury.[51] Such individuals should be referred to an ophthalmologist for complete evaluation and clearance.

Finally, abnormal visual acuity is among the most frequently reported findings during the PPE.[2,6,9,11] Athletes who are identified as having abnormal visual acuity at the time of the PPE should be evaluated and treated by an eyecare professional.

GYNECOLOGIC DISORDERS AND PREGNANCY

Because ovarian injury is so unlikely in sports, no restrictions are necessary for female athletes with only 1 ovary. Athletes with menstrual disorders should receive a complete evaluation by a physician. Such individuals should also be screened for signs of disordered eating and a history of stress fractures.[45,47,48] A nutritional evaluation to assess the adequacy of caloric intake relative the athlete's energy expenditure should be considered.[46-48] Athletes with oligomenorrhea or amenorrhea usually may be cleared while undergoing further evaluation. If pregnancy is suspected, clearance for contact-collision or strenuous sports participation should be withheld pending either a negative pregnancy test or clearance by the clinician who is following the pregnancy. The need for routine gynecologic care in an asymptomatic individual (eg, Pap smear) is not a reason to deny or delay clearance.

HEAT ILLNESS (RECURRENT)

The athlete with a history of heat illness may be at risk for recurrent heat illness.[52,53] Because these athletes may have unique characteristics that affect their ability to acclimate to hot environments, they need further assessment to determine the presence of predisposing conditions and to arrange a prevention strategy. Meticulous monitoring of the training environment, gradual acclimatization, and the gradual introduction of vapor-barrier equipment can help to reduce the risk. Tracking individual fluid losses, and proper fluid and electrolyte replacement, are essential to preventing cumulative dehydration. Recurrent heat illness may also be due to a medical condition, such as obesity or febrile illness; medications, such as antihistamines, antidepressants, psychomotor stimulants; or poor physical conditioning.[54]

The presence of sickle cell trait should be considered in athletes with a history of heat illness, because such individuals may be at greater risk for heat illness, including heatstroke, and may be at risk for sickling during exertion in the heat or at altitude.[55-59] It is plausible that, in individuals with sickle cell trait, dehydra-

tion—due to an inability to fully concentrate the urine—increases the risk of heat illness. However, confusion exists between sickling collapse and heatstroke. It appears that some deaths attributed to heatstroke may actually have been due to sickling.[55,59]

Although clearance need not be denied to athletes with a history of heat illness, a specific prevention strategy should be implemented. Athletes with sickle cell trait, even if they have no history of heat illness, should receive specific counseling regarding the prevention of sickling during exertion. Athletes with a documented history of heatstroke or heat-related rhabdomyolysis also merit further investigation. Clearance for these athletes should be individualized.

HEPATOMEGALY AND SPLENOMEGALY

Organomegaly is a cause for concern if there is increased risk of damage to the organ or malfunction of a vital organ. The underlying cause must also be determined.

Acute hepatomegaly may signal the presence of infection (eg, hepatitis, infectious mononucleosis [mono]) or malignant disease (eg, hepatocellular carcinoma, lymphoma). A liver that is enlarged beyond the bony protection of the rib cage is at risk of injury. Even though the incidence of hepatic rupture among patients with acute hepatomegaly is low, participation in all sports should be avoided. Full activity may be resumed after resolution of hepatomegaly.

An athlete who has acute splenomegaly should not participate in sports. This situation is most frequently encountered in the athlete diagnosed with infectious mono. Athletes with the condition should be restricted from participation because of the rare, but serious, complication of splenic rupture.[60,61] Furthermore, because splenic rupture in mono can occur in the absence of trauma, athletes should be restricted from all forms of sports-related activity.[60,61] Determining when it is safe to return the athlete recovering from mono to sports is based on the resolution of clinical symptoms and the risk for splenic rupture.

Once symptoms have resolved, the decision to resume activity is difficult, since there are no prospective studies available that have assessed the spleen. The greatest risk for splenic rupture in those with infectious mono is within the first 21 days of illness in those with splenic enlargement.[60] Splenic rupture very rarely occurs beyond 28 days, but it has been reported.[62]

Complicating the return-to-play decision is that, although acute splenomegaly commonly develops, the physical examination cannot be relied on to determine its presence.[63] Serial ultrasound examination of the spleen in these patients, however, indicates that spleen size appears to normalize within 28 days.[63] Based on these data, athletes with mono should be restricted from all sports-related activities for the first 21 days of illness. (If the date of symptom onset is not known, the date of the diagnosis should be used as the starting point.) If the patient is asymptomatic by day 21, light activities can be undertaken for the 4th week, with full participation resumed at week 5. Some clinicians employ serial ultrasound measurements as an additional tool in determining return to play. However, it may be difficult to determine when the spleen size has normalized, because parameters for spleen size based on gender, height, weight, and ethnicity have not yet been established and may vary considerably among individuals.[64]

For individuals with chronic hepatomegaly or splenomegaly, participation in sports should be assessed individually and decisions based on the degree of enlargement and the associated disease state.

INGUINAL HERNIA

An athlete with an asymptomatic inguinal hernia may participate in all sports. Symptomatic inguinal hernias may limit an athlete's ability to participate and may be affected by activity. Such symptomatic cases invariably require treatment at some time and should be evaluated individually.

KIDNEY ABNORMALITIES

Because of the potential for kidney injuries ranging from contusion to complete rupture, special consideration should be given when determining clearance for an athlete who has a single functioning kidney. Some, but not all, experts believe that if the kidney is pelvic, iliac, or multicystic, or shows evidence of hydronephrosis or ureteropelvic junction abnormalities, the athlete should not participate in contact-collision sports. The consequences of the loss of a single functioning kidney (eg, transplantation or dialysis) may be severe enough to warrant disqualification from these sports, even though the risk is small.[65] Evaluation by a urologist or nephrologist is recommended.

If the athlete chooses to play in a sport that may place a solitary kidney at increased risk for damage, a full explanation should be given to the athlete, his or her parent(s) or guardian(s), and the coaches. The explanation should include available protection (eg, flak jacket), potential serious long-term consequences, and treatment of injuries if they occur.

MUSCULOSKELETAL DISORDERS

Determining clearance for athletes who have musculoskeletal injuries or disorders requires assessing both short- and long-term risks and benefits, considering carefully the general questions on page 61. Clearance for participation must be based on the degree and type of injury, the ability of the injured athlete to compete safely, and the requirements of a given sport. Participation may be possible in activities that do not directly affect the injured site (eg, a wrist sprain might prevent a gymnast from full training, but not a runner). Therefore, the physician should also determine which strength and conditioning activities are appropriate during the recovery period so that the athlete is able to maintain some level of fitness.

Protective padding, taping, or bracing may be designed to provide the athlete a safe means to compete. The types of protective splinting or bracing permitted in competition varies by the sport and the rules of the sport organization or league. If the examining physician is not certain of the rules concerning safe participation with protective devices, consultation with a sports medicine specialist is suggested. The final decision on what type of protective padding or bracing to use may rest with the on-site officials. In such situations, a change in the original type of protection recommended by the sports medicine staff could be deemed necessary by the official. Any alteration required by the official should be evaluated to ensure that it provides the necessary protection for the injury.

Referral to a consultant is warranted when the examiner is uncertain of the athlete's ability to participate because of the injury. In any case, physicians who initiated the treatment of an injury that was present at the time of the PPE should be included in the clearance decision. Reevaluation is required after rehabilitation.

Review of every musculoskeletal problem is beyond the scope of this monograph, but selected problems deserve mention:

Sprains, subluxations, and dislocations. Before clearance is given, sprains, subluxations, and dislocations should be examined and the following ruled out:

◆ Effusion, swelling, or other signs of inflammation;

◆ Decreased range of motion of the affected joint;

◆ Strength less than 85% to 90% of the uninjured side or insufficient for the desired activity;

◆ Ligamentous instability of the affected joint; and

◆ Loss or alteration of sport-specific functional ability (ie, inability to complete pain-free functional activity at 100% effort). For example, a football defensive back who is rehabilitating a lateral ankle sprain could be assessed with back-pedaling and side-to-side movements.

If any of these findings are abnormal, further treatment will be needed to allow for return to play. Referral, if necessary, to a physician familiar with the sport-specific requirements and injury assessment is recommended. Ultimately, the decision for clearance is based on the examiner's clinical judgment and may be withheld until further evaluation and completion of prescribed treatment or rehabilitation. Further evaluation and appropriate consultation is warranted if uncertainty about clearance persists.

Strains or muscle contusions. Before clearance is given, strains or muscle contusions should be examined and the following ruled out:

◆ Decreased range of motion of joints controlled by the muscle;

◆ Strength less than 85% to 90% of the uninjured side or insufficient for the desired activity; and

◆ Loss or alteration of sport-specific functional ability.

Treatment and clearance decisions parallel those for sprains, subluxations, and dislocations (above).

Overuse injuries. Overuse or overload injuries are caused by repetitive microtrauma. Examples include stress fractures, Achilles tendonopathy, medial and lateral epicondylitis, plantar fasciitis, patellofemoral pain syndrome, rotator cuff tendonopathy, and impingement syndrome. Clearance decisions are generally based on criteria similar to those for acute sprains or strains.

Fractures. Clearance of an athlete with a fracture should be determined by the treating physician. The location and type of fracture, risk of reinjury or complications, and the effect of treatment should be con-

sidered. The possibility of protecting the fracture with a cast or splint during participation should be considered if the risk of worsening the injury is believed to be negligible. Also, in making clearance decisions, the physician should be aware of specific rules relevant to the athlete's sport regarding use of padded and unpadded materials on the extremities. Contacting a league representative or referral to a sports medicine specialist is warranted if the examiner or treating physician is unfamiliar with options regarding protective devices.

Developmental conditions. Any history or physical findings of spinal deformity (eg, scoliosis, spondylolysis, or spondylolisthesis) require a more thorough evaluation than is generally provided in the PPE. Follow-up with the athlete's primary care physician, sports medicine specialist, or spine specialist is recommended should questions arise. Spondylolysis and spondylolisthesis should be evaluated individually on the basis of symptoms, physical limitations, and imaging findings. Because of the risk of progressive slippage, spondylolysis or spondylolisthesis may require follow-up imaging. Generally, athletes with spinal deformities need not be excluded from play. However, activities may need to be modified based on clinical symptoms and the extent of the abnormality.

Clearing athletes who have apophysitis of the tibial tubercle (Osgood-Schlatter disease), calcaneus (Sever's disease), ileum, or ischium follows similar criteria as for overuse injuries and acute strains.

If there are any questions concerning clearance, sports medicine consultation is suggested.

◼ NEUROLOGIC DISORDERS

Careful assessment of the neurologic history is important in determining clearance for athletes who have a history of concussion or other head injury, burners or stingers, or seizure disorders.

Concussion. The most common serious head injury in contact-collision sports is the cerebral concussion, also termed mild traumatic brain injury. An estimated 300,000 such injuries occur annually in the United States.[66]

Although the definition of concussion is not universally agreed upon, the First International Symposium on Concussion in Sport recently defined concussion as a complex pathophysiologic process affecting the brain, induced by traumatic biomechanical forces.[67]

This consensus group described several characteristic features that further enhance the definition[67]:

◆ Concussion may be caused either by a direct blow to the head, face, neck, or by a blow elsewhere on the body with an "impulsive" force transmitted to the head. Concussion typically results in the rapid onset of short-lived impairment of neurologic function that resolves spontaneously.

◆ Concussion may result in neuropathologic changes, but the acute clinical symptoms largely reflect a functional disturbance rather than structural injury.

◆ Concussion results in a graded set of clinical syndromes that may or may not involve loss of consciousness. Resolution of the clinical and cognitive symptoms typically follows a sequential course.

◆ Concussion is typically associated with grossly normal structural neuroimaging studies.

There are multiple concussion classification and management protocols in the literature, based primarily on clinical experience and expert opinion.[68] The complexity of concussion and the lack of large outcome studies have hampered the development of evidenced-based management recommendations. Recent studies using symptom checklists and neuropsychological testing have begun to describe the natural history of sports-related concussion.[69,70] Such studies demonstrate the importance of the monitoring of clinical symptoms and the potential value of neuropsychological testing in concussion management.[68,69,71] Furthermore, athletes with a history of concussion appear to be at higher risk of future concussion, and those with a history of multiple concussions may suffer long-term sequelae.[71-73]

Athletes at the PPE who report a history of a recent concussion should be individually assessed to ensure symptom resolution and to determine an appropriate level of activity. Symptomatic individuals should not be cleared for participation. Any physician determining return to play following a concussion should be familiar with the current literature and commonly referenced clinical recommendations. Because of the present lack of evidenced-based guidelines, such decisions ultimately are made based on the clinical judgement of the physician.

Those with a history of concussion who have been asymptomatic should be educated on the signs and symptoms of concussion and encouraged to report the occurrence of such symptoms. Baseline neuropsycho-logical testing may be considered in athletes with a history of concussion to provide an additional tool in the management of future concussions. The role of baseline neuropsychological testing for participants with no history of concussion who are competing in high-risk sports such as football, soccer, and ice hockey is an area of emerging research.[74-76]

"Second impact syndrome." A rare but catastrophic entity has been described in which diffuse cerebral edema develops after head trauma. This injury has been reported primarily in children and teenagers, and at times has occurred after minimal head trauma.

The mechanism of injury is thought to involve disruption of cerebral vascular autoregulation, with resultant brain swelling and increased intracranial pressure causing high morbidity and mortality. It has been proposed that this syndrome is precipitated by head trauma that occurs when symptoms of a prior concussion or head injury are still present or by repeated concussions and has therefore been termed second impact syndrome.[77,78] However, it has recently been questioned whether this injury occurs as a result of previous head trauma or simply occurs due to a single impact.[79]

Burners and stingers. Athletes who have had an episode of transient neurapraxia affecting an upper extremity, commonly termed a "burner" or "stinger," may be cleared for all sports if they are asymptomatic and their physical examination is normal. Athletes with a history of recurrent episodes or persisting symptoms following a single episode, require evaluation with cervical spine radiographs and additional imaging to rule out a predisposing condition such as cervical disk disease, foraminal stenosis, or cervical spinal stenosis.

Transient quadriparesis. Athletes with a history of transient quadriparesis (sometimes referred to as cervical spinal cord neurapraxia) should be evaluated by a spine subspecialist. Those who have had an episode of transient quadriparesis and who have findings of ligamentous instability, cord injury or edema, or prolonged symptoms should be excluded from participation in contact sports.[80,81] For all other athletes with a history of transient quadriparesis, including those with congenital or acquired cervical spinal stenosis, return to play is controversial.[80-83]

Seizure disorder. Athletes with a treated and controlled seizure disorder can participate in nearly all sports. Sports or activities that entail high risk (eg, gymnastics on high apparatus, high diving, skydiving, motor sports, rock climbing) should be avoided.[84,85] When athletes have poorly controlled seizures, clearance should be deferred for contact-collision, limited-contact, and potentially hazardous noncontact sports, such as archery, riflery, swimming, weight lifting or power lifting, strength training, or sports involving heights.[13] In the interim, while medications are adjusted and seizure control is improving, athletes may participate in noncontact sports that do not involve risk to themselves or others. In the rare instance that athletic activity precipitates an athlete's seizures, clearance should be denied and the athlete referred to a neurologist.

OBESITY

Childhood obesity has reached epidemic proportions.[86] Physicians performing the PPE will undoubtedly encounter athletes who are obese, and concerns may arise as to whether to clear them. Although individuals with obesity may have associated conditions (eg, hypertension, EIA, susceptibility to heat injury, diabetes, slipped capital femoral epiphysis), there is no reason to exclude them from sports participation because of their weight alone.

In fact, once underlying causes of obesity have been ruled out (eg, thyroid deficiency), every effort should be made to encourage some type of sports participation. Such athletes, however, should receive counseling on specific strategies to prevent heat-related illnesses. Any associated medical conditions must be appropriately treated and monitored.

PHYSICAL MATURITY STATUS

Concerns may arise regarding clearance of an adolescent who is relatively delayed in physical maturation or underweight and who seeks to participate in competitive sports. There is no medical reason to exclude such an individual from sports participation unless a coexisting condition warrants exclusion.

PULMONARY DISORDERS

The most prevalent pulmonary problem in athletes is exercise-induced bronchoconstriction (EIB). The term EIB is usually used in referring to those who have symptoms (eg, shortness of breath, wheezing, chest

tightness, cough) that occur during or after exercise and who do not have a history of asthma.[87] EIA refers to patients with a diagnosis of asthma who have exercise-related symptoms. The prevalence of EIB is highest among those who compete in cold-weather sports.[88]

Arriving at a diagnosis of EIB can be difficult, especially since self-reported symptoms poorly predict the condition.[89] During the PPE, physicians should evaluate athletes who report symptoms consistent with EIB. In addition, those who report EIB should have their records reviewed to ensure that an accurate diagnosis was made. It is important to determine that the exercise-associated symptoms are not simply the most apparent manifestation of chronic asthma. Therefore, spirometry to document the patient's forced expiratory volume in 1 second (FEV_1) should be performed.

For those with a history consistent with EIB and a normal FEV_1 on spirometry, a presumptive diagnosis of EIB may be made, and a therapeutic trial of medication can be instituted, along with instructions for a preexercise warm-up. The medication most often used is a beta-agonist taken by inhalation. It is important for the clinician to ensure that the athlete is using the inhaler correctly.

Provocational testing is necessary to confirm the diagnosis of EIB when it is in doubt or for those in whom a therapeutic trial does not improve function. *Challenge testing may also be necessary to establish documentation for medication use in national and international competitions.* The type of challenge test that best diagnoses EIB has not been established. Examples include field-based exercise testing, laboratory-based exercise testing, methacholine challenge testing, eucapnic voluntary hyperventilation, and osmotic challenge tests.[87]

Finally, it is rarely necessary to withhold an athlete with EIB or chronic asthma from participation in sports, although appropriate treatment is necessary to ensure optimal performance. Athletes whose PPE findings are suggestive of EIB or asthma may participate while being treated and monitored by a physician as their evaluation is being completed.

TESTICULAR DISORDERS

The incidence of testicular injury in sports is extremely low.[90] An individual with a single testicle may be cleared for participation, with the use of a protective cup for higher-risk sports.[13] However, the athlete with a solitary testicle who wishes to participate in contact-collision sports must be informed that there is a risk of injury and loss of the testicle. Although wearing a protective cup may reduce the incidence of injury, it does not guarantee complete protection. Protective cups can be cumbersome and uncomfortable, and some athletes prefer not to wear them. However, with a thorough explanation of the potential benefits and availability of more comfortable cups, many athletes will choose to wear protection to decrease their risk of injury. In addition, the athlete with

a solitary testicle who chooses to compete in sports should be informed of the option of sperm banking to preserve fertility and its associated costs should an injury to the testicle occur.

If an athlete has an undescended testicle that has not been thoroughly evaluated, the examining physician should refer him for evaluation and inform him of the increased risk of testicular cancer associated with this condition. Clearance determination for an athlete who has an undescended testicle is similar to that for an athlete with a single testicle.

REFERENCES

1. Linder CW, DuRant RH, Seklecki RM, et al: Preparticipation health screening of young athletes: results of 1268 examinations. Am J Sports Med 1981;9(3):187-193
2. Goldberg B, Saraniti A, Witman P, et al: Pre-participation sports assessment—an objective evaluation. Pediatrics 1980;66(5):736-745
3. Thompson TR, Andrish JT, Bergfeld JA: A prospective study of preparticipation sports examinations of 2670 young athletes: method and results. Cleve Clin Q 1982;49(4):225-233
4. Tennant FS Jr, Sorenson K, Day CM: Benefits of preparticipation sports examinations. J Fam Pract 1981;13(2):287-288
5. Magnes SA, Henderson JM, Hunter SC: What conditions limit sports participation? Experience with 10,540 athletes. Phys Sportsmed 1992;20(5):143-160
6. Risser WL, Hoffman HM, Bellah GG Jr: Frequency of preparticipation sports examinations in secondary school athletes: are the University Interscholastic League guidelines appropriate? Tex Med 1985;81(7):35-39
7. DuRant RH, Seymore C, Linder CW, et al: The preparticipation examination of the athlete. Comparison of single and multiple examiners. Am J Dis Child 1985:139(7):657-661
8. Rifat SF, Ruffin MT 4th, Gorenflo DW: Disqualifying criteria in a preparticipation sports evaluation. J Fam Pract 1995:41(1):42-50
9. Smith J, Laskowski ER: The preparticipation physical examination: Mayo Clinic experience with 2,739 examinations. Mayo Clin Proc 1998;73(5):419-429
10. Lively MW: Preparticipation physical examinations: a collegiate experience. Clin J Sport Med 1999;9(1):3-8
11. DiFiori JP, Haney S: Preparticipation evaluation of collegiate athletes. Med Sci Sports Exerc 2004;36(5 suppl):S102
12. Stevens MB, Smith GN: The preparticipation sports assessment. Fam Pract Recert 1986;8(3):68-88
13. Committee on Sports Medicine and Fitness, American Academy of Pediatrics: Medical conditions affecting sports participation. Pediatrics 107(5):1205-1209
14. 26th Bethesda Conference: Recommendations for determining eligibility for competition in athletes with cardiovascular abnormalities. January 6-7, 1994. Med Sci Sports Exerc 1994;26(10 suppl):S223-283 [published erratum appears in Med Sci Sports Exerc 1994;26(12): following table of contents]
15. Mitchell JH, Haskell WL, Raven PB: Classification of sports. Med Sci Sports Exerc 1994;26(10 suppl):S242-S245
16. Green GA,Catlin DH, Starcevic B: Analysis of over-the-counter dietary supplements. Clin J Sport Med 2001:11(4):254-259
17. Scott MJ, Scott MJ Jr: HIV infection associated with injections of anabolic steroids. JAMA 1989;262(2):207-208
18. Aitken C, Delalande C, Stanton K: Pumping iron, risking infection? Exposure to hepatitis C, hepatitis B and HIV among anabolic-androgenic steroid injectors in Victoria, Australia. Drug Alcohol Depend 2002;65(3):303-308
19. Torre D, Sampietro C, Ferraro G, et al: Transmission of HIV-1 infection via sports injury. Lancet 1990;335(8697):1105
20. Brown LS Jr, Drotman DP, Chu A, et al: Bleeding injuries in professional football: estimating the risk for HIV transmission. Ann Intern Med 1995;122(4):273-274
21. Committee on Sports Medicine and Fitness , American Academy of Pediatrics: Human immunodeficiency virus and other blood-

borne viral pathogens in the athletic setting. Pediatrics 1999; 104(6):1400-1403
22. Kashiwagi S, Hayashi J, Ikematsu H, et al: An outbreak of hepatitis B in members of a high school sumo wrestling club. JAMA 1982; 248(2):213-214
23. Ringertz O, Zetterberg B: Serum hepatitis among Swedish track finders: an epidemiologic study. N Engl J Med 1967; 276(10):540-546
24. Moyer LA, Mast EE, Alter MJ: Hepatitis C: Part 1, routine serologic testing and diagnosis Am Fam Physician 1999;59(1):79-92
25. Human immundeficiency virus and other blood-borne pathogens in sports. The American Medical Society for Sports Medicine (AMSSM) and the American Academy of Sports Medicine (AASM). Clin J Sport Med 1995;5(3):199-204
26. 2003-04 NCAA Sports Medicine Handbook, pp 36-40. Available at http://www.ncaa.org/library/sports_sciences/sports_med_handbook/2003-04/. Accessed July 15, 2004
27. Chobanian AV, Bakris GL, Black HR, et al: Seventh report of the Joint National Committee on Prevention, Detection, Evaluation, and Treatment of High Blood Pressure. Hypertension 2003;42(6):1206-1252. Epub 2003 Dec, 01. Available at http://www.nhlbi.nih.gov/guidelines/hypertension/. Accessed August 26, 2004
28. National Heart, Lung, and Blood Institute: Blood pressure tables for children and adolescents from the Fourth Report on Diagnosis, Evaluation, and Treatment of High Blood Pressure in Children and Adolescents. Available at http://www.nhlbi.nih.gov/guidelines/hypertension/child_tbl.htm. Accessed July 15, 2004
29. Maron BJ: Sudden death in young athletes. N Engl J Med 2003; 349(11):1064-1075
30. Corrado D, Basso C, Schiavon M, et al: Screening for hypertrophic cardiomyopathy in young athletes. N Engl J Med 1998;339(6): 364-369
31. Maron BJ, McKenna WJ, Danielson GK, et al: American College of Cardiology/European Society of Cardiology clinical expert consensus document on hypertrophic cardiomyopathy: a report of the American College of Cardiology Foundation Task Force on Clinical Expert Consensus Documents and the European Society of Cardiology Committee for Practice Guidelines. J Am Coll Cardiol 2003;42(9):1687-1713
32. Estes NA 3rd, Link MS, Cannom D, et al, Expert Consensus Conference on Arrhythmias in the Athlete of the North American Society of Pacing and Electrophysiology: Report of the NASPE policy conference on arrhythmias and the athlete. J Cardiovasc Electrophysiol 2001;12(10):1208-1219
33. 2003-04 NCAA Sports Medicine Handbook, p 21. Available at http://www.ncaa.org/library/sports_sciences/sports_med_handbook/2003-04/. Accessed July 15, 2004
34. Anderson BJ: The epidemiology and clinical analysis of several outbreaks of herpes gladiatorum. Med Sci Sports Exerc 2003; 35(11):1809-1814
35. Anderson BJ: The effectiveness of valacyclovir in preventing reactivation of herpes gladiatorum in wrestlers. Clin J Sport Med 1999;9(2):86-90
36. Methicillin-Resistant *Staphylococcus aureus* infections among competitive sports participants: Colorado, Indiana, Pennsylvania, and Los Angeles County, 2000-2003. MMWR 2003;52(33):793-795

37. Mines BA, Nguyen D, DiFiori JP, et al: Factors associated with CA-MRSA outbreak among collegiate athletes. Poster presentation, American Medical Society for Sports Medicine annual meeting, Vancouver, BC, April 19, 2004

38. National Federation of State High School Associations: Wrestling Sports/Rules Information. Available at http://www.nfhs.org/scriptcontent/va_Custom/va_Cm/newspage.cfm?Category_ID=36&Content_ID=195&showarchive=No&itemtitle=Item&Title=Wrestling%20Sports%20Information&head=WR.cfm. Accessed August 26, 2004

39. 2004 NCAA Wrestling Rules and Interpretations: Appendix D: Skin infections. Indianapolis, IN, National Collegiate Athletic Association, 2004. Available at http://www.ncaa.org/library/rules/2004/2004_wrestling_rules.pdf. Accessed August 26, 2004

40. Birrer RB, Sedaghat V-D: Exercise and diabetes mellitus: optimizing performance in patients who have type 1 diabetes. Phys Sportsmed 2003;31(5):29-41

41. Bhaskarabhatla KV, Birrer RB: Physical activity and type 2 diabetes: tailoring exercise to optimize fitness and glycemic control. Phys Sportsmed 2004;32(1):13-17

42. Zinman B, Ruderman N, Campaigne BN, et al: American Diabetes Association Position Statement: Diabetes mellitus and exercise. Diabetes Care 2002;25:S64

43. Draznin MB: Type 1 diabetes and sports participation: strategies for training and competing safely. Phys Sportsmed 2000;28(12):49-56

44. Tsui EY, Chiasson JL, Tildesley H, et al: Counterregulatory hormone responses after long-term continuous subcutaneous insulin infusion with lispro insulin. Diabetes Care 1998;21(1):93-96

45. Otis CL, Drinkwater B, Johnson M, et al: American College of Sports Medicine position stand: The female athlete triad. Med Sci Sports Exerc 1997;29(5):i-ix

46. Loucks AB, Verdun M, Heath EM: Low energy availability, not stress of exercise, alters LH pulsatility in exercising women. J Appl Physiol 1998;84(1):37-46

47. Nattiv A: Stress fractures and bone health in track and field athletes. J Sci Med Sport 2000;3(3):268-279

48. De Souza MJ, Williams NI: Physiological aspects and clinical sequelae of energy deficiency and hypoestrogenism in exercising women. Hum Reprod Update 2004;10(5):433-448

49. American Academy of Pediatrics Committee on Sports Medicine and Fitness: Protective eyewear for young athletes. Pediatrics 2004;113(3 pt 1):619-22

50. Napier SM, Baker RS, Sanford DG, et al: Eye injuries in athletics and recreation. Surv Ophthalmol 1996;41(3):229-244

51. Rodriguez JO, Lavina AM, Agarwal A: Prevention and treatment of common eye injuries in sports. Am Fam Physician 2003;67(7):1481-1488

52. Armstrong LE, De Luca JP, Hubbard RW: Time course of recovery and heat acclimation ability of prior exertional heatstroke patients. Med Sci Sports Exerc 1990;22(1):36-48

53. Epstein Y: Heat intolerance: predisposing factor or residual injury? Med Sci Sports Exerc 1990;22(1):29-35

54. 2003-04 NCAA Sports Medicine Handbook, pp 22-24. Available at http://www.ncaa.org/library/sports_sciences/sports_med_handbook/2003-04/. Accessed July 15, 2004

55. Pretzlaff RK: Death of an adolescent athlete with sickle cell trait caused by exertional heat stroke. Pediatr Crit Care Med 2002;3(3):308-310

56. Kerle KK, Nishimura KD: Exertional collapse and sudden death associated with sickle cell trait. Am Fam Physician 54(1):237-240

57. Kark JA, Ward FT: Exercise and hemoglobin S. Semin Hematol 1994;31(3):181-225

58. Martin TW, Weisman IM, Zeballos RJ, et al: Exercise and hypoxia increase sickling in venous blood from an exercising limb in individuals with sickle cell trait. Am J Med 1989;87(1):48-56

59. Wirthwein DP, Spotswood SD, Barnard JJ, et al: Death due to microvascular occlusion in sickle-cell trait following physical exertion. J Forensic Sci 2001;46(2):399-401

60. Maki DG, Reich RM: Infectious mononucleosis in the athlete: diagnosis, complications, and management. Am J Sports Med 1982;10(3):162-173

61. Farley DR, Zietlow SP, Bannon MP, et al: Spontaneous rupture of the spleen due to infectious mononucleosis. Mayo Clin Proc 1992;67(9):846-853

62. Johnson MA, Cooperberg PL, Boisvert J, et al: Spontaneous splenic rupture in infectious mononucleosis: sonographic daignosis and follow-up. Am J Roentgenol 1981;136(1):111-114

63. Dommerby H, Stangerup SE, Stangerup M, et al: Hepatosplenomegaly in infectious mononucleosis, assessed by ultrasonic scanning. J Laryngol Otol 1986;100(5):573-579

64. Hosey R: Spleen size in athletes: a comparison of gender and race. Presented at the American Medical Society for Sports Medicine Annual Meeting, April 19, 2004, Vancouver, BC

65. Sharp DS, Ross JH, Kay R: Attitudes of pediatric urologists regarding sports participation by children with a solitary kidney. J Urol 2002;168(4 pt 2):1811-1814

66. Thurman DJ, Branche CM, Sniezek JE: The epidemiology of sports-related traumatic brain injuries in the United States: recent developments. J Head Trauma Rehabil 1998;13(2):1-8

67. Aubry M, Cantu R, Dvorak J, et al, Concussion in Sport Group: Summary and agreement statement of the First International Conference on Concussion in Sport, Vienna 2001. Phys Sportsmed 2002;30(2):57-63

68. McKeag DB: Understanding sports-related concussion: coming into focus but still fuzzy. JAMA 2003;290(19):2604-2605

69. McCrea M, Guskiewicz KM, Marshall SW, et al: Acute effects and recovery time following concussion in collegiate football players: the NCAA Concussion Study. JAMA 2003;290(19):2556-2563

70. Collins MW, Iverson GL, Lovell MR, et al: On-field predictors of neuropsychological and symptom deficit following sports-related concussion. Clin J Sport Med 2003;13(4):222-229

71. Collins MW, Grindel SH, Lovell MR, et al: Relationship between concussion and neuropsychological performance in college football players. JAMA 1999;282(10):964-970

72. Guskiewicz KM, McCrea M, Marshall SW, et al: Cumulative effects associated with recurrent concussion in collegiate football players: the NCAA Concussion Study. JAMA. 2003;290(19):2549-2555

73. Rabadi MH, Jordan BD: The cumulative effect of repetitive concussion in sports. Clin J Sport Med 2001;11(3):194-198

74. Lovell MR: The relevance of neuropsychologic testing for sports-related head injuries. Curr Sports Med Rep 2002;1(1):7-11

75. Schatz P, Zillmer EA: Computer-based assessment of sports-related concussion. Appl Neuropsychol 2003;10(1):42-47

76. Lovell M, Collins M, Bradley J: Return to play following sports-related concussion. Clin Sports Med 2004;23(3):421-441

77. Saunders RL, Harbaugh RE: The second impact in catastrophic contact-sports head trauma. JAMA 1984;252(4):538-539

78. Cantu RC, Voy R: Second impact syndrome: a risk in any contact sport. Phys Sportsmed 1995;23(6):27-34

79. McCrory P: Does second impact syndrome exist? Clin J Sport Med 2001;11(3):144-149

80. Torg JS: Cervical spinal stenosis with cord neurapraxia: evaluation and decisions regarding participation in athletics. Curr Sports Med Rep 2002;1(1):43-46

81. Fagan K: Transient quadriplegia and return-to-play criteria. Clin Sports Med 23(3):409-419

82. Castro FP Jr: Stingers, cervical cord neurapraxia, and stenosis. Clin Sports Med 2003;22(3):483-492

83. Cantu RC: Cervical spine injuries in the athlete. Semin Neurol 2000;20(2):173-178

84. Fountain NB, May AC: Epilepsy and athletics. Clin Sports Med 2003;22(3):605-616, x-xi

85. Dubow JS, Kelly JP: Epilepsy in sports and recreation. Sports Med 2003;33(7):499-516

86. Ogden CL, Flegal KM, Carroll MD, et al: Prevalence and trends in overweight among US children and adolescents, 1999-2000. JAMA 2002;288(14):1728-1732

87. Holzer K, Brukner P: Screening of athletes for exercise-induced bronchoconstriction. Clin J Sport Med 2004;14(3):134-138

88. Storms WW: Review of exercise-induced asthma. Med Sci Sports Exerc 2003;35(9):1464-1470

89. Rundell KW, Im J, Mayers LB, et al: Self-reported symptoms and exercise-induced asthma in the elite athlete. Med Sci Sports Exerc 2001;33(2):208-213

90. McAleer IM, Kaplan GW, LoSasso BE: Renal and testis injuries in team sports. J Urol 2002;168(4 pt 2):1805-1807

Chapter 8
THE ATHLETE WITH SPECIAL NEEDS

A thletes with special needs (physical and intellectual disabilities) represent a growing population of sports participants. Federal legislation mandating equal access and equal opportunity to physical education and sports for persons with special needs as well as extraordinary accomplishments by athletes with special needs have ignited this growth.[1]

The Americans With Disabilities Act defines a disability as an impairment that limits a major life activity.[2] Types of disabilities include cerebral palsy, blindness, deafness, paralysis, mental retardation, and amputation, as well as locomotor disabilities such as arthritis, muscular dystrophy, and multiple sclerosis.

BENEFITS OF SPORTS

Sports participation for athletes with special needs provides the same benefits as for athletes without special needs: increased exercise endurance, muscle strength, and flexibility; improved cardiovascular function, balance, and motor skills; and psychological benefits, including increased self-esteem, reduced anxiety and depression, and the satisfaction derived from participation and competition. In addition, some benefits from sports participation are unique to the athlete with special needs (table 26).[3]

PPE FOR SPECIAL NEEDS

The PPE for the athlete with special needs should be similar to that of an athlete without a physical or intellectual disability. In addition, the PPE should address the particular concerns of the athlete with special needs. The healthcare provider should be aware of common problems associated with different disabili-

ties and be able to diagnose abnormalities that may endanger the athlete. Just as important, the healthcare provider should provide support and encourage physical activity.

Athletes with special needs are classified according to the severity of their disability. To promote fairness in competition, athletes with similar degrees of disability compete against one another (for more details on this aspect, see "Administrative and Legal Concerns," chapter 4, page 11).

The Special Olympics and the United States Paralympics, a division of the United States Olympic Committee, have organized sports events for athletes with special needs.

Special Olympics is an international organization dedicated to empowering individuals 8 years old and older with intellectual disabilities to become physically fit through sports training and competition.[4] Special Olympics offers year-round training and competition in 26 summer and winter sports.

Special Olympics currently serves more than 1 million people who have intellectual disabilities in more than 200 programs in more than 150 countries. In 2000, Special Olympics made a bold commitment to reach 2 million athletes by the end of 2005. This means that more physicians will encounter increasing numbers of Special Olympians who will seek PPEs and sports-related medical and surgical care.

The Special Olympics are arranged at local, state, and international levels, and participation requires a PPE.[5] Depending on the state or level of competition, the PPE needs to be performed every 1 to 3 years. Special Olympics World Games, for example, require a PPE to be performed within 12 months of a competition.

United States Paralympics features more than 20 sponsored sports and provides funding and facilities for persons with physical disabilities.[6] The Paralympic Games are held every Olympic year and provide competitions for more than 5,000 athletes with physi-

Table 26	Benefits of Sports Participation Unique to Those With Special Needs (Compared With Inactive Counterparts)	
Athletes With Paraplegia		**Athletes With Amputations**
Fewer pressure ulcers		Improved proprioception
Fewer infections		Increased proficiency using
Lower likelihood of hospitalization		prosthetic devices

cal disabilities in Summer and Winter Games. New technology applied to prosthetic devices allows increasingly more physically impaired athletes to participate at higher levels of competition.

METHODS OF EVALUATION

The office-based PPE is preferred to the station-based or mass screening examination. The decreased mobility of some athletes with special needs makes the station method less practical. The PPE should be performed by a healthcare provider involved in the longitudinal care of the athlete as described in "Timing, Setting, and Structure," chapter 3 (page 5). Specialty consultations are sometimes necessary.

THE PPE MEDICAL HISTORY

As in the general PPE guidelines, a thorough medical history is essential to an informed participation recommendation. The history form should be completed by the athlete (if possible) and parents or guardian familiar with the athlete's medical history. In addition, a parent or guardian may need to be present at the time of the PPE in order to obtain the most accurate answers to questions. This is especially true for athletes participating in the Special Olympics.

The history should include a detailed summary of previous injuries and illnesses, risk factors for injuries and illnesses, and current medications.

Questions. In addition to the questions asked of an athlete without a physical or intellectual disability (see "The PPE Medical History," chapter 5, page 17, and the history form, page 93), questions in the history of an athlete with a special need should be individualized and address the particular disability. The questions that follow emphasize areas of greatest concern for sports participation:

1. Does the athlete have a history of seizures, hearing loss, or vision loss? Are the seizures controlled? These are common abnormalities seen in Special Olympic athletes.[7] Uncontrolled seizures often require a consultation with a neurologist and a delay in clearing the athlete for sports participation.

2. Does the athlete have a history of cardiopulmonary disease? Congenital cardiac disorders, including heart murmurs, ventricular septal defects, and endocardial cushion defects, are more common in persons with Down syndrome.

3. Does the athlete have a history of renal disease or unilateral kidney? Various renal anomalies, such as hypoplasia, dysplasia, and obstruction, are more common in people with Down syndrome.[8]

4. Does the athlete have a history of atlantoaxial instability? Spontaneous or traumatic subluxation of the cervical spine is a potential risk in athletes with Down syndrome.[9]

5. Has the athlete had heatstroke or heat exhaustion? Thermoregulation in athletes with spinal cord injuries is impaired because of skeletal muscular paralysis and a loss of autonomic nervous system control. Medications used for pain and bladder dysfunction can interfere with the normal sweat response. Also, athletes who have had a history of heat illness are more prone to again develop the condition.

6. Has the athlete had any fractures or dislocations? Ligamentous laxity and joint hypermobility are prominent features in athletes with Down syndrome.

7. What prosthetic devices or special equipment does the athlete use during sports participation? Healthcare providers need to be aware of an athlete's need for adaptive equipment and regulations concerning their use in different sports.

8. Does the athlete use an indwelling urinary catheter or require intermittent catheterization of the bladder? Athletes with spinal cord injuries or other neurologic disorders often have bladder dysfunction or neurogenic bladders.

9. Does the athlete have a history of pressure sores or ulcers? Athletes who use wheelchairs are prone to pressure ulcers at the sacrum and ischial tuberosities, and athletes who use prostheses are prone to pressure ulcers at prosthesis sites.

10. At what levels of competition has the athlete previously participated?

11. What is the athlete's level of independence for mobility and self-care?

12. What medications is the athlete taking?

13. Is the athlete on a special diet?

14. Does the athlete have a history of autonomic dysreflexia? This is an acute, potentially life-threatening syndrome of excessive, uncontrolled sympathetic output that can occur in athletes with spinal cord injuries at or above the sixth thoracic spinal cord level.[10] This reflex may happen spontaneously or may be self-induced ("boosting") by an athlete in an attempt to improve performance.[11]

Triggers for autonomic dysreflexia include bowel or bladder distension, infections (especially of the urinary tract), sunburn, ingrown toenails, and wearing tight garments.

Signs and symptoms of autonomic dysreflexia include excessively high blood pressure, a pounding headache, sweating above the level of spinal injury, flushed face, and bradycardia.

Boosting is a dangerous performance-enhancing technique that is strictly forbidden by all sports governing bodies. Athletes with spinal cord injuries at T-6 or above sometimes use this technique in an effort to improve cardiopulmonary performance, oxygen utilization, and noradrenaline release. Methods of boosting include occluding one's own urinary catheter and ingesting large amounts of fluids prior to an event to extend the bladder.[3]

◣ THE PPE PHYSICAL EXAMINATION

The PPE physical examination for the athlete with a special need should include all parts of the examination as for the athlete without a physical or intellectual disability (see "The PPE Physical Examination," chapter 6, page 45, and the physical examination form, page 94). Particular attention should be given to the visual, cardiovascular, musculoskeletal, neurologic, and dermatologic systems (table 27).

In addition to examining the athlete, healthcare providers should thoroughly inspect all prostheses, orthoses, and assistive or adaptive devices to ensure adequate construction for sports participation and proper fit.[12]

Vision. Eye examinations of Special Olympic athletes reveal a high prevalence of vision abnormalities. A study[13] of Special Olympics athletes at the 1995 International Summer Games revealed that almost one third of the athletes had ocular problems. The most common problems identified were poor visual acuity, refractive errors, astigmatism, and strabismus.

Cardiovascular system. Congenital heart disease is present in as many as 50% of athletes with Down syndrome.[14] Many of these athletes may require further testing (eg, ECG, echocardiogram) or clearance from a cardiologist before participating in sports. Decisions for further testing or consultation should follow the same guidelines as for the athlete without a disability.

Table 27	**Findings to Screen for When Performing Physical Examinations on Athletes With Special Needs**

Vision
Poor visual acuity
Refractive errors
Astigmatism
Strabismus

Cardiovascular System
Congenital heart disease

Neurologic System
Peripheral nerve entrapment
    Carpal tunnel syndrome
    Ulnar neuropathy (Guyon's tunnel syndrome)
Inadequate motor control
Inadequate coordination and balance
Impaired hand-to-eye coordination
Ataxia
Muscle weakness
Fatigue
Spasticity
Sensory dysfunction
Atlantoaxial instability
Hyperreflexia
Clonus
Upper motor neuron and posterior column
    signs and symptoms

Dermatologic System
Abrasions
Lacerations
Blisters
Pressure ulcers
Rashes

Musculoskeletal System
Limited neck range of motion
Torticollis
Decreased flexibility, often with contractures,
    decreased strength, and muscle strength
    imbalance

Neurologic system. Since many athletes with special needs have some form of neurologic deficit, a complete neurologic evaluation should be performed.

Peripheral nerve entrapment syndromes of the upper extremities are common in wheelchair athletes. Two of the most common entrapment syndromes are carpal tunnel syndrome and ulnar neuropathy at the wrist (Guyon's tunnel syndrome). The examiner should look for signs of muscle atrophy and weakness in the hand and sensory deficits following a specific nerve distribution. He or she should perform provocative tests such as Tinel's sign over the median and ulnar nerves in the wrist.

Athletes with cerebral palsy frequently have inadequate motor control and lack adequate coordination and balance for participation in different sports. Hand-to-eye coordination is also impaired. Evaluating these functions will reveal whether sports requiring catching, throwing, and controlling necessary equipment such as floor hockey sticks, rackets, and bats will be difficult or even dangerous to the athlete or other competitors.

Athletes with multiple sclerosis have varying degrees of disability. The examiner should check for ataxia, muscle weakness, fatigue, spasticity, and sensory dysfunction.

Approximately 15% of children with Down syndrome have atlantoaxial instability.[15] A very small number of these children develop signs and symptoms of cervical cord myelopathy. The neurologic manifestations of symptomatic atlantoaxial instability include easy fatigue, abnormal gait, incoordination and clumsiness, sensory deficits, spasticity, hyperreflexia, clonus, and other upper motor neuron and posterior column signs and symptoms.

Dermatologic system. Athletes in wheelchairs are especially prone to skin injuries. The upper extremities should be examined for abrasions and blisters caused by friction, shear, and irritation from repeated contact with the wheelchair push rim. Skin wounds can also result from contact with other chairs, wheelchair brakes, or sharp edges of the wheelchair.

The skin over the sacrum and ischial tuberosities should be inspected for pressure ulcers. Athletes in wheelchairs have elevated skin pressures in these regions for prolonged periods during training, competition, and normal daily activity. Sports wheelchairs are designed so that the athlete's knees are at a higher level than the buttocks, a position that leads to increased pressure over the sacrum and ischial tuberosities.[1] During sports participation, the combination of skin pressure, shear, and moisture increases the risk for pressure ulcers. Athletes in wheelchairs who have a pressure ulcer should not be cleared for sports participation until there is complete healing of the wound. The chair seat should be modified to decrease the risk of future skin trauma.

Prostheses can cause skin trauma; the prosthesis site should be inspected for abrasions, blisters, rashes, and pressure ulcers. The presence of pressure ulcers precludes participation in sports until the condition has resolved. The prosthesis should be evaluated for proper fit and reconditioned to decrease the risk of future problems. In the skeletally immature athlete, overgrowth of the stump can be a problem leading to breakdown of the overlying skin and soft tissues.[11]

Genitourinary system. Examination should involve the same evaluation as for athletes without a disability, as well as any external devices used for bladder drainage.

Musculoskeletal system. The musculoskeletal examination of an athlete who uses a wheelchair should include evaluation of the stability, flexibility, and strength of commonly injured sites (eg, shoulder, hand, and wrist) and the trunk.[3]

Athletes with lower limb amputation and prostheses require a full assessment of the lower back and lower extremities. These are common areas of injury resulting from abnormal forces and motions placed during sports activities.

Musculoskeletal manifestations of atlantoaxial instability in athletes with Down syndrome include limited range of motion of the neck and torticollis or head tilt. Because of hypermobility and ligamentous laxity, athletes with Down syndrome have an increased incidence of hip and knee injuries.[14] Examination may reveal signs of instability and weakness.

Athletes with cerebral palsy have decreased musculotendinous flexibility, often with contractures, decreased strength, and muscle strength imbalances—especially of the lower extremities—that vary in severity from mild and nearly imperceptible to very severe and wheelchair bound.[1] Overuse injuries, strains, and sprains are common, especially at the hips, knees, ankles, and feet. The PPE should include a thorough examination of these regions.

FUNCTIONAL ASSESSMENT

An individualized functional assessment of all athletes with special needs should be part of the PPE. An athlete's overall mobility while using prosthetic, orthotic, assistive, or adaptive devices should be evaluated. Sport-specific tasks should also be incorporated into the evaluation. A physical therapist with expertise in the area can assist with this portion of the evaluation.

DIAGNOSTIC IMAGING

Athletes with symptomatic atlantoaxial instability should have cervical spine radiographic imaging to assess the extent of the problem. Radiographs of the lateral cervical spine with flexion and extension views assess the space between the posterior aspect of the anterior arch of the atlas and the odontoid.

Even though there is no evidence confirming the value of these radiographs in asymptomatic athletes with Down syndrome and atlantoaxial instability, the Special Olympics requires that athletes with Down syndrome competing in certain sports and events have a radiologic evaluation for atlantoaxial instability. The events for which such a radiologic examination is required are: judo, equestrian sports, gymnastics, diving, pentathlon, butterfly stroke and diving starts in swimming, high jump, Alpine skiing, snowboarding, squat lift, and soccer.[16]

DETERMINING CLEARANCE

Clearance for sports participation should follow the same principles as for athletes without physical or intellectual disabilities (see "Determining Clearance," chapter 7, page 61). Healthcare providers need to assess the safety of a given sport for an athlete with special needs. The athlete's medical condition and functional abilities, and the demands of the sport, need to be taken into account.

Athletes with atlantoaxial instability should be restricted from sports that require excessive neck flexion or extension.[15] See above (under "Diagnostic Imaging") for a list of those sports.

Pressure sores are common occurrences in athletes using prostheses or wheelchairs.[17] Athletes with pressure sores should not be cleared for sports participation until there is complete healing at the involved sites.

REFERENCES

1. Halpern BC, Cardone DA: The athlete with a disability, in Safran MR, McKeag DB, Van Camp SP (eds): Manual of Sports Medicine. Philadelphia, Lippincott-Raven, 1998, pp 190-198
2. Nichols AW: Sports medicine and the Americans with Disabilities Act. Clin J Sport Med 1996;6(3):190-195
3. Malanga GA, Filart R, Cheng J: Athletes with disabilities. Available at http://www.eMedicine.com/sports/topic144.htm. Accessed July 16, 2004
4. Information for Special Olympics available at http://www.specialolympics.org. Accessed July 16, 2004
5. Mooar PA: Experiences as sports coordinator for the Philadelphia County Special Olympics. Clin Orthop 2002; 396 (Mar):50-55
6. Information for US Paralympics. Available at http://www.usparalympics.org. Accessed August 19, 2004
7. McCormick DP, Ivey FM Jr, Gold DM, et al: The preparticipation sports examination in Special Olympics athletes. Tex Med 1988;84(4):39-43
8. Mercer ES, Broecker B, Smith EA, et al: Urological manifestations of Down syndrome. J Urol 2004;171(3):1250-1253
9. Committee on Sports Medicine, American Academy of Pediatrics: Atlantoaxial instability in Down Syndrome. Pediatrics 1984;74(1):152-154
10. Blackmer J: Rehabilitation medicine: 1. Autonomic dysreflexia. CMAJ 2003;169(9):931-935
11. Boosting and Autonomic Dysreflexia, in International Paralympic Committee Handbook. Bonn, Germany, 2002, section II, chapter 8
12. Patel DR, Greydanus DE: The pediatric athlete with disabilities. Pediatr Clin North Am 2002;49(4):803-827
13. Block SS, Beckerman SA, Berman PE: Vision profile of the athletes of the 1995 Special Olympics World Summer Games. J Am Optom Assoc 1997;68(11):699-708
14. Winell J, Burke SW: Sports participation of children with Down syndrome. Orthop Clin North Am 2003;34(3):439-443
15. Committee on Sports Medicine and Fitness, American Academy of Pediatrics: Atlantoaxial instability in Down syndrome: subject review. Pediatrics 1995;96(1 pt 1):151-154
16. Application for Participation in Special Olympics. United States Special Olympics,2004. Available from Special Olympics, 1325 G St NW, Ste 500, Washington, DC 20005. More information at http://www.specialolympics.org. Accessed July 16, 2004
17. Dec KL, Sparrow KJ, McKeag DB: The physically-challenged athlete: medical issues and assessment. Sports Med 2000;29(4):245-258

Chapter 9

FUTURE CONSIDERATIONS FOR PREPARTICIPATION EXAMS

Because the PPE is the only routine primary or preventive healthcare many students receive,[1] future consideration should be given to a core exam that can be expanded not only to meet the needs of the athlete but to improve the PPE process. Even the best exams lack sufficient sensitivity to consistently recognize clinically important anomalies in the athlete. There are no scientific data to support how best to screen for medical problems or how to stratify the risk for short- and long-term health problems prior to sports participation. The most important element in the conventional PPE—the medical history—is often inadequate. In addition, the validity of the questions used in medical screening is unknown.

The current examination is not tailored to specific populations or age-groups. Considerable variability exists in the screening from state to state and most likely from physician to physician, and the exam oversimplifies what should be a more detailed and targeted screening process. Liability has increased for schools, associations, athletic trainers, administrators, and coaches because of health-related issues stemming from sports participation. Finally, liability risk to physicians has increased as questions arise about the thoroughness of the screening process.

KEY DIRECTIONS
Future considerations for the PPE should include: (1) working toward a common accepted format, if not a single form; (2) multicenter, randomized comparisons of the frequency of the exam to determine optimal recommendations; and (3) databases to measure effectiveness and validity of the PPE process.

Common form. A common form ideally should approach the Institute of Medicine's (IOM's) concept of core exam components. However, even the recommended questions in this monograph have not been validated for wording, completeness, or sufficiency and efficiency in addressing risks. Development and adoption of a common form that applies to all PPE settings nationwide will be a challenging and evolving process.

Optimal frequency. Before we decide on the most appropriate frequency, we must first have evidence that a given one is superior, and gathering such data will be important in shaping the future PPE. Healthcare delivery itself may influence timing. Patients are mobile, insurance coverage changes, and team physicians change.

Measuring the PPE's effectiveness. Clearly, we need to know if our screening affects outcome. Future study design will likely require reliance on large databases that are not currently available. Electronic medical recording of the PPE may point the way.

ELECTRONIC OPPORTUNITIES
All of the changes to the PPE process as outlined in this monograph set the stage for continued reevaluation. The IOM has questioned the value of the traditional "annual physical." Nationally, the need for standardized, mandatory screening has received much attention. Can we make the PPE more than the screening exam it was intended to be?

Innovative use of Internet technology may provide an expedient and thorough method of screening for sports and exercise. This was the conclusion of a study based at Stanford University[2] that described the development and implementation of a Web-based PPE used on Stanford varsity athletes. The authors used a questionnaire to collect comprehensive medical history data. Physicians then used a computer-generated summary to focus the physical exam. Researchers found good compliance and acceptance, improved exam efficiency, and strong subjective satisfaction with the quality of screening provided.

In addition, use of the Internet may allow capture of relevant medical information that could be tracked and tested over time to improve the performance of the exam and the efficacy of the questions. Policy recommendations to govern safe participation in sports have not been based on an overall understanding of issues and conditions that affect athletes. Incorporating an electronic medical record into the PPE process may allow positive exam findings to be targeted with expanded questions and examination findings using embedded devices like drop-down boxes and nested branched-chain questions. This process would allow even the less experienced examiner to focus on what is important for each athlete without missing key questions. Electronic methodology also lends to expansion of the basic exam for those with sport-specific interests and for research purposes without changing the basic screening format.

The goals of an ideal electronic PPE (e-PPE) are to support the frontline physician, who must make rational and defensible decisions for sports participation, by developing and implementing a tool that:

◆ Emphasizes and facilitates a detailed comprehensive history;

◆ Provides the mechanism to standardize and simplify the screening process for physicians;

◆ Provides a screening process that is tailored to sport, age, population, and sex;

◆ Is easy to administer and use;

◆ Is relatively inexpensive;

◆ Allows the athlete to choose any physician to perform the exam and receive a comparable result;

◆ Provides a data set for risk factor identification;

◆ Maintains confidentiality and security of student-athlete medical information consistent with the Health Insurance Portability and Accountability Act (HIPAA) of 1996; and

◆ Allows surveillance and trends information to direct improvements in athletic care.

Electronic information management. In early 2003, the American Health Information Management Association (AHIMA) appointed a task force of experts to develop a vision of the electronic health information management (e-HIM) future. The task force stated: "The future state of health information is electronic, patient-centered, comprehensive, longitudinal, accessible, and credible." To promote the recommendations of the e-HIM Task Force, AHIMA created working groups to develop practice standards that focus on areas that play an integral role in the transition from paper to electronic health records.[3] This transition will no doubt improve the PPE process.

But managing health information in a hybrid environment is challenging, particularly given the requirements of managing the transition.[3] A hybrid health record includes both paper and electronic documents and may smooth the path.

The PPE described in this monograph lends itself to incorporating the medical information questions in an electronic version. This format simplifies the

process for the majority who have not had health problems and allows a focus on what is important for the athlete with positive medical or family history or positive physical findings. Advantages may vary among the different ways in which this could be implemented.

Two possible solutions for improving the PPE are both technically feasible and available: (1) an e-PPE and (2) a paper-to-electronic format.

▶ ELECTRONIC PPE PILOT PROJECT

An electronic method for acquiring medical information conceivably offers a much better way to screen for medical problems that increase the risk for sports and exercise. When combined with a summary report generated for the screening physician, this approach provides an excellent method for collecting the most important data.

The Stanford study stimulated interest in and facilitated development of a Web-based e-PPE that emphasizes the importance of a comprehensive medical history to identify at-risk athletes. Its health history questionnaire replaces or augments current forms. Each student completes his or her own secure health history, from which a physician's summary and required participation forms are generated. The e-PPE does not affect the way schools conduct their preparticipation screening. It is appropriate to use in either office- or station-based physicals.

To develop the comprehensive questionnaire for the e-PPE, a software design company worked in partnership with an international team, including sports medicine physicians from Stanford University, the University of Calgary, and members of the Joint Advisory Committee on Sports Medicine of the Ohio State Medical Association and the Ohio High School Athletic Association.

Based on a literature search that identified more than 500 references, 260 references were determined to be relevant for detailed review using evidence-based medicine. To ensure due diligence and rigor, these references were used to create an inclusive list of questions, followed by epidemiologic analysis to arrive at a draft set of optimal questions. The draft questions were subjected to peer review and consensus evaluation by a conference of physicians and licensed athletic trainers. Recommendations for revision were made, and questions were again modified.

In addition, other material was collected to further support the due diligence process. All states were surveyed to learn about their current processes, and questionnaires currently used were collected. The questionnaires and forms were compared with questions and forms being created for the e-PPE.

The result of this research was a comprehensive 75-item branched-chain questionnaire that incorporated validated subscales and addressed the areas of greatest concern to the health of student-athletes, including cardiovascular disease, cervical spine instability, absence of paired vital organs, and weight-bearing joint instability. The final questionnaire was then incorporated as a key component of the Web-based e-PPE.

Security. Confidentiality was considered paramount, and multiple measures were taken to ensure privacy of all information on the questionnaire. Proven security measures were used:

◆ Password protection;

◆ Secure sockets layer-encryption;

◆ Results database kept separate from personal profile; and

◆ Firewall-secured server site with data backup, intrusion detection, and access controls.

Access to the e-PPE was limited to the student through a self-selected user name and password. Only the student, parents, and physicians saw the summary that was printed with the answers to the questionnaire. Authorization to release the answers or any medical information obtained through the questionnaire could be given only by the students and/or parents or guardians.

Students' questionnaire answers were never linked directly to their identity. Under no circumstances was access allowed or granted to their personal contact information. All information was transmitted to the server using a secure sockets layer-encryption technology. The database storing information resided on a physically separate server that was not accessible directly from the Internet, further protecting the data from unauthorized access. When students saved their information, it was transmitted to servers over the Internet in encrypted form. All student personal contact information was kept in encrypted form in a separate database from the answers they provided when completing a questionnaire. The IP (Internet Protocol) address of a computer was stored, but it was used only to create broad demographic summaries of user location. Security statements were developed for students, parents, and administrators to help alleviate any concerns.

Electronic questionnaire. The e-PPE begins with a comprehensive online health history questionnaire for each student-athlete. The student logs on to the e-PPE Web site before the physical examination. There is no software to install on the computer. The student answers questions on such issues as current and past medical problems, injuries, family and medical history, medications, allergies, and eating habits. Depending on the responses to key questions, more detailed information may be requested using nested, branched-chain questions.

Students can answer all the questions in one sitting or log off and come back as needed to complete the questionnaire. Parents should always be involved in the health history. Once students complete all 12 sections of the questionnaire, they are instructed to print out all the supplied forms.

Summary and physical exam. A relevant summary of the answers is generated from the questionnaire, printed by the student, and handed to the physician or medical examiner during the preparticipation physical exam. This summary highlights any conditions that may affect safe sports participation. The examiner then makes a clearance decision based on the detailed information on the student's e-PPE summary and physical exam findings. The students' e-PPEs are stored so that only updates and significant changes are required in subsequent years, which decreases the time spent filling out the questionnaire.

Forms. The e-PPE provides all necessary printed forms and releases for parents, students, and physicians to sign. These include the consent to participate, emergency information, medical history summary, and physical exam forms. Upon completion of the physical examination, the physician completes the form titled "Consent to Participate in School Sports" and assigns the student to 1 of 4 categories: (1) cleared to participate with no restrictions, (2) cleared to participate with the following restrictions (as detailed), (3) deferred—may reconsider after further evaluation, or (4) not cleared to participate: not fit. The consent to participate and the emergency information forms are returned to the athletic administrator. The medical history summary and physical examination form remain with the examining physician.

Of greatest significance to physicians is the medical history summary that extracts relevant details about the student's health and family history from the questionnaire database and condenses the history into an easy-to-review printed summary. Both positive and pertinent negative responses are included. This 2- to 3-page synopsis allows the physician to immediately identify conditions that should be considered when evaluating a student for sports participation. This simplifies the physical examination process for the physician. The physician is not required to enter any data, and the medical history summary enables a focused physical examination. A complete printout of the history is also available. The extra level of detail provided by the e-PPE may take a little more time for the physician to assimilate, but this extra time is offset by the ability of the summary to focus attention on the specific health issues of each student.

Tracking tools. A tool for school athletic administrators allows them to track and record the progress of the students through the e-PPE questionnaire, create status reports of athletes, generate team reports, and—once the physical examination is complete—keep a record of the athlete's participation clearance. The athletic administrator tool is automatically populated with student information as the students register to use the e-PPE. The list of students can be sorted or filtered by a number of criteria, such as their sport, school grade, gender, or clearance status. This tool allows athletic administrators to monitor the eligibility of athletes yearly. No student is inadvertently left out.

The athletic trainer or high school activities or athletic director can also use the tool to log clearance status. Any restrictions or conditions noted by the examining physician can be entered. This capability would enable any sports administrator at the school to easily determine changes in clearance of any student-athlete at the school throughout the year.

Assessing the project. A pilot program was conducted to assess the effectiveness of the e-PPE and included 28 Ohio high schools and more than 4,400 students.[4] Feedback was gathered from students, parents, athletic administrators, and physicians.

Feedback from students and parents was predominantly positive. Negative feedback centered on length, amount of detail, and resistance to change. Completion time averaged 45 minutes but improved with experience, 70% of students involved their parents, 96% fully understood what they were required to do, 80% believed it was easy to use, 29% sought help from within the program (of these, 60% readily found the help needed), and 68% agreed that the program was better in collecting important medical information than traditional PPE forms.

Reaction of participating athletic administrators was overwhelmingly positive. About 77% of schools saw merit and would participate, but the magnitude of the technology hurdle was a consideration for some. Physicians responded favorably. The medical history summary was perceived as very thorough and was particularly helpful for physicians who were not sports medicine specialists. The information enabled physicians to interact with the students in a more meaningful way. By requiring the students to answer all questions and by having parents help the students to answer the questionnaire, the physicians gained more complete information at the time of the examination.

Medical information from the pilot program revealed several important findings. For more than 55% of student-athletes, the preparticipation screening was the only physical examination they received. Previously unreported epidemiologic data was documented. The incidence of certain conditions was just as frequent in the student-athlete population as in the nonathlete population (for example, asthma was found in 10% of both populations). Potentially significant conditions occurred in the student-athlete more frequently than thought. For example, self-reporting revealed that 10% had a history of concussion, 12% had restrictions in the past, 2% had serious eye injuries, and 3% were without 2 normally functioning kidneys.

Preliminary data analysis revealed a surprising number of positive responses to questions related to significant risk factors, such as cardiovascular and heat-related illness. Seventy percent had positive answers to cardiovascular screening questions, 8.5% had a family history of cardiovascular death before age 50, and 23% reported dizziness during and after exercise. This high number of positive responses to these segments of the questionnaire suggests that the current nationally accepted questions might not be appropriate to detect cardiovascular problems in this population.

Possible health risk behaviors were reported frequently. For example, 18.5% were carefully controlling weight, and 5% used pathologic weight-control methods. There were a number of unresolved problems from sports-related injuries (for example, 1% had residual symptoms of concussion, and 1% had unresolved neck injury). Medication and supplement use were common: Prescription medications were used by 21%, more than 1 prescription medication by 6%, nonprescription medications by 32%, and supplements by 15%.

Financing. Funding options for this or a similar program included the following possibilities: (1) each school would pay an annual fee per athlete, (2) corporate sponsors would be recruited, (3) cost of championship tickets would be increased to cover the cost, and (4) less expensive programs with readily available software would be developed.

Effective overall. Despite the hurdles in implementing a new program, the e-PPE demonstrated its ability to identify athletes who require further evaluation, which enhances the health and safely of the athletes. Findings from the e-PPE highlight the need to educate all physicians involved with student-athletes.

PAPER-TO-ELECTRONIC APPROACH

Those who perform the PPE should be prepared to make the transition to an electronic health record (EHR). On July 1, 2003, the secretary of the US Department of Health and Human Services (HHS), Tommy Thompson, announced that the department is moving the healthcare industry toward implementation of the EHR. He announced that HHS had commissioned the IOM to design a standardized model of an EHR. The model record has not been published as this monograph goes to press but most likely will include core data sets similar to those in the current PPE.[5] Any group designing an electronic form should consider 3 important issues: (1) conversion of the present PPE form to one that can be managed electronically and/or placed on a secured Web site, (2) development of a form that allows multiple uses and multiple means of access, and (3) use of form-design software that can interface with database programs to provide query resources for all contributors. Query resources allow investigators to set up queries to deal with their particular research interests and then retrieve information from the common database.

One approach might be to convert the current PPE forms to electronic forms that could be placed on the Web sites of each state's high school league or association (or other governing authority for eligibility) so that all schools could either: (1) make multiple paper copies for athletes and families to fill out at home; (2) start allowing athletes to answer history questions directly on the Internet via sites that are either maintained by a software producer, protected at the state health department, or under state athletic authority; or (3) scan paper forms back into electronic file using optical recognition. Although paper poses more difficult issues under HIPAA, it is the most likely vehicle to smoothly bring parents from the old to the new system and to fit into the transition occurring in the offices of physicians who are administering the exam.

CONSIDERATIONS FOR ELECTRONIC IMPLEMENTATION

There are advantages and disadvantages to using an electronic approach (table 28). Considerations need to include software design, database interface, information security, data management, and research facilitation.

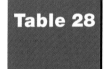

Table 28 Advantages and Disadvantages of Electronic Handling of Athletic Health Information

Advantages
Better data management
Built-in research capabilities
Easily modifiable to incorporate new information
Can be expanded without changing basic screening format
Facilitation of security and privacy
Interfacing database programs for specific query
Ready integration of new evidence-based medicine into the PPE process

Disadvantages
Expensive transitions
Need for educating users
Time commitment
Changing technologies, software, and hardware
Dependence on technical expertise

User-friendly software design. Forms should be compatible with other EHR systems to facilitate transfer of information.[6] Typical configurations can allow selective sharing of information. This allows "must know" information to be available but protects components that should not be shared:

◆ *User profiles* (name and demographics of athlete) would be a separate form, linked to history and physical findings by social security number and self-selected user name or password combination. Profiles would contain eligibility information for state athletic authority and schools, emergency contact information, background information for insurance claims, physician offices and referrals, and classification of athletes' clearance status.

◆ *Individual medical record* (secured for HIPAA and the 1974 Family Education Rights and Privacy Act [FERPA]) would be available to medical personnel involved with the care of the individual athlete, to authorized persons under emergency situations, and for research purposes.

◆ *Injury record* would be programmed to accept ongoing data entry for prospective surveillance. It would be used for improving the history, targeting the physical exam, and identifying the type, anatomic site, and severity of past injuries. It would allow new injury information to be added from hospital discharges and emergency department visits, including those covered under Medicaid or state health plans.

Each component must contain stand-alone information that addresses the interests of all contributors and be interrelated with the complete medical record but anonymous in its isolated form.

An interface with database programs. In the past, athletic injury or occurrence data has been gathered in labor-intense and often skewed fashion. Facilitating access to multiple databases with information that either enhances the depth of each separate database or acts as a check-and-balance system for accuracy should be considered when software is chosen. The ability to obtain retrospective and prospective data is possible with the surveillance of ongoing athletic health information. Possibilities include: (1) eligibility and demographic data that can be shared with school administrations and high school leagues or associations, (2) medical information that can be shared with physicians' offices, (3) injury surveillance applications compatible with all of above and able to accept sport

specific data, (4) information about player participation hours and level of competition from other databases, and (5) core data sets like those HHS has commissioned the IOM to design.

Security and privacy. Security can be ensured with carefully designed systems. Considerations include sufficient safeguards to ensure:

◆ Viewing of messages by their intended recipients only;

◆ Verification of delivery and receipt;

◆ Labeling of sensitive material;

◆ Control of access by those other than the provider; and

◆ Security of computer hardware and software.

Browser-based communication with patients has advantages, because it provides additional security as compared with e-mail. For example, users are required to log in, and audit trails are accessible. Security/encryption, physical security, structured messaging, approval/revocation options, and access (group vs single) are more characteristic of browser-based communication.

Data management. Sufficiently extensive data can be collated to allow an individually performed exam to carry the same weight as each exam performed in a large uniform protocol when integrated into a data pool. The PPE content can be rapidly updated, which creates a living document for all users. Problems of different languages can be minimized by electronic conversion between languages. The ability to integrate interim history and injury information will allow transition to entry-level exams with a history update. This should help decrease the annual burden on healthcare resources.

Research capability. Another advantage of the e-PPE is the ability to generate research in additional areas such as the public health, including the previously discussed epidemiologic considerations. Generation of forms for the healthcare team from the PPE not only facilitates communication but also enables further refining of data input needed for evidence-based research. Examples might be an emergency information form, a return-to-play form, injury surveillance, and sport-specific health concerns.

Using this "tag-on" research will allow better evaluation and study of the PPE process to confirm its validity, specificity, and sensitivity.[2] The outcomes of athletes with prior injury, health risks, obesity, conditioning deficiencies, and other factors could be assessed and interventions evaluated. Larger databases, incidence and exposure data for sports-related injuries, improved surveillance and communication, research opportunities, and refinement of the PPE instrument itself will substantiate the value of the exam.

The expansive and standardized collection of medical history information provides an opportunity to study factors associated with risk of disease and injury in student athletes. A yearly analysis of the aggregated data could concentrate on two key indicators: (1) high-prevalence responses that point out common, but usually less serious findings and (2) low-prevalence or rare responses that point to more severe conditions or those known to carry significant public health impact.

This type of process allows the collection of important information about the student-athlete population as a whole. Examination of the data collected provides an opportunity to conduct detailed studies, approved by internal review boards, that may lead to a true understanding of the prevalence of preexisting conditions. Interventions can be recommended to reduce health risk before participation in sports. Risk profiles for athletes would evolve as more data are collected and studied. Once analysis reveals areas of concern, health screening and health programs within schools can be established to target these areas. Yearly analysis

of the data will provide the best opportunity to create an environment for the student-athletes that simultaneously balances concerns for short- and long-term health with maximizing performance in competitive sports.

FUTURE TRANSITIONS

The PPE process offers an excellent opportunity to promote the recommendations of the e-HIM Task Force and to develop practice standards that focus on areas that play an integral role in the transition from paper to electronic health records. Application of electronic methodology to the PPE will mirror the IOM's ideal of a standardized model of an EHR. Sensitivity, specificity, validity, application to a specific population, and new information gained can and should be used to profile risk to a large, somewhat homogeneous population. Starting this process with young athletes is justified because: (1) we have a defined, albeit captive, population to study, (2) we are addressing concerns of an even larger exercising public, and (3) athletes are exposed to substantial increases in metabolic and physical load.

We should try to achieve the standards of rigor in preventive healthcare delivery that medicine in general tries to achieve. Therefore, future direction will reflect more than just the needs of our young athletes.

REFERENCES

1. American Academy of Pediatrics Web site. Available at www.aap.org. Accessed July 19, 2004
2. Peltz JE, Haskell WL, Matheson GO: A comprehensive and cost-effective preparticipation exam implemented on the World Wide Web. Med Sci Sports Exerc 1999;31(12): 1727-1740
3. American Health Information Management Association: Electronic Health Information Management (eHIM). Available at http://library.ahima.org/xpedio/groups/public/documents/ahima/pub_bok1_021580.html. Accessed July 19, 2004 (Reader should refer to the entire collection of recommendations to best understand transitions.)
4. Wingfield KW, Matheson GO, Meeuwisse WH:

Preparticipation evaluation: an evidence-based review. Clin J Sport Med 2004;14(3):109-122
5. American Health Information Management Association: AHIMA e-HIM Work Group on Core Data Sets for the Physician Practice Electronic Health Record (AHIMA Practice Brief): Core data sets: pediatric well patient clinical work flow: new patient and established patient. Available at http://library.ahima.org/xpedio/groups/public/documents/ahima/pub_bok1_021607.html. Accessed July 19, 2004
6. American Health Information Management Association: AHIMA e-HIM Work Group on Electronic Document Management as a Component of the Electronic Health Record: Available at http://library.ahima.org/xpedio/groups/public/documents/ahima/pub_bok1_021599.html. Accessed July 19, 2004

The PPE is ideally done as a part of routine health screening examinations by an athlete's primary physician. If integrating the exam into periodic health screening is not possible, a PPE involving multiple examiners in private screening areas can be employed. The group exam format can be optimized by using 1 physician to do the entire history review, exam, and clearance statement for each athlete.

With one third of young athletes leaving sports by age 13,[1] and many youth sports leagues not requiring a PPE for participation, young patients should be asked, as a part of their health screening exams, if they participate in or intend to participate in youth sports. If the answer is yes, the questions from the PPE become an integral part of the health screening exams for the patient. If the answer is no, the encounter should be used to encourage physical activity, and the same questions critical to the PPE should be addressed.

Although the PPE should be done about 6 weeks before the season begins, in reality, many of the exams are done at the "11th hour" and do not leave time for evaluation of suspicious or abnormal findings before sports practice begins. Physicians must be firm in completing the full evaluation of any positive findings from the screening exam before allowing athletes to participate. Athletes need to be educated to have the exams conducted in a timely manner. The Institute for Clinical Systems Improvement recommends periodic health screening in those older than 5 years at ages 7, 9, 12, 15, and 18,[2] which blends well with the suggested PPE frequency.

The physician-athlete interaction associated with the PPE may serve as the foundation for a trusting relationship, help optimize the athlete's long-term health, and, for many healthy adolescent athletes, be their only contact with the healthcare system. Young athletes should know that the exam is in their best interest and will be conducted entirely confidentially.

With a thorough evaluation and knowledgeable counseling, physicians and other healthcare professionals can use the PPE as an opportunity to enhance the safety of sports participation and promote a healthy lifestyle. The PPE can provide a "teachable moment" that is not always available to teenage athletes who are often involved in high-risk activities away from the playing field. As a whole, the exam should promote safe, cost-effective athletic participation while providing a springboard for healthy behaviors during the risky adolescent years and throughout life.

REFERENCES

1. Wolff A: The American athlete, age 10: time of their lives or too much too soon? Sports Illustr 2003;99(14):59-67
2. ICSI Pocket Guidelines, April 2004. Bloomington, MN, Institute for Clinical Systems Improvement, 2003

Preparticipation Physical Evaluation

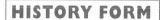

HISTORY FORM

DATE OF EXAM_____

Name_____	**Sex**_____ **Age**_____ **Date of birth**_____
Grade____ **School**_____	**Sport(s)**_____
Address_____	**Phone**_____
Personal physician_____	

In case of emergency, contact

Name_____ **Relationship**_____ **Phone (H)**_____ **(W)**_____

Explain "Yes" answers below.
Circle questions you don't know the answers to.

                                              Yes No

1. Has a doctor ever denied or restricted your participation in sports for any reason? ☐ ☐
2. Do you have an ongoing medical condition (like diabetes or asthma)? ☐ ☐
3. Are you currently taking any prescription or nonprescription (over-the-counter) medicines or pills? ☐ ☐
4. Do you have allergies to medicines, pollens, foods, or stinging insects? ☐ ☐
5. Have you ever passed out or nearly passed out DURING exercise? ☐ ☐
6. Have you ever passed out or nearly passed out AFTER exercise? ☐ ☐
7. Have you ever had discomfort, pain, or pressure in your chest during exercise? ☐ ☐
8. Does your heart race or skip beats during exercise? ☐ ☐
9. Has a doctor ever told you that you have (check all that apply):
   ☐ High blood pressure   ☐ A heart murmur
   ☐ High cholesterol   ☐ A heart infection
10. Has a doctor ever ordered a test for your heart? (for example, ECG, echocardiogram) ☐ ☐
11. Has anyone in your family died for no apparent reason? ☐ ☐
12. Does anyone in your family have a heart problem? ☐ ☐
13. Has any family member or relative died of heart problems or of sudden death before age 50? ☐ ☐
14. Does anyone in your family have Marfan syndrome? ☐ ☐
15. Have you ever spent the night in a hospital? ☐ ☐
16. Have you ever had surgery? ☐ ☐
17. Have you ever had an injury, like a sprain, muscle or ligament tear, or tendinitis, that caused you to miss a practice or game? If yes, circle affected area below: ☐ ☐
18. Have you had any broken or fractured bones or dislocated joints? If yes, circle below: ☐ ☐
19. Have you had a bone or joint injury that required x-rays, MRI, CT, surgery, injections, rehabilitation, physical therapy, a brace, a cast, or crutches? If yes, circle below: ☐ ☐

Head	Neck	Shoulder	Upper arm	Elbow	Forearm	Hand/ fingers	Chest
Upper back	Lower back	Hip	Thigh	Knee	Calf/shin	Ankle	Foot/toes

20. Have you ever had a stress fracture? ☐ ☐
21. Have you been told that you have or have you had an x-ray for atlantoaxial (neck) instability? ☐ ☐
22. Do you regularly use a brace or assistive device? ☐ ☐
23. Has a doctor ever told you that you have asthma or allergies? ☐ ☐

                                                              Yes No

24. Do you cough, wheeze, or have difficulty breathing during or after exercise? ☐ ☐
25. Is there anyone in your family who has asthma? ☐ ☐
26. Have you ever used an inhaler or taken asthma medicine? ☐ ☐
27. Were you born without or are you missing a kidney, an eye, a testicle, or any other organ? ☐ ☐
28. Have you had infectious mononucleosis (mono) within the last month? ☐ ☐
29. Do you have any rashes, pressure sores, or other skin problems? ☐ ☐
30. Have you had a herpes skin infection? ☐ ☐
31. Have you ever had a head injury or concussion? ☐ ☐
32. Have you been hit in the head and been confused or lost your memory? ☐ ☐
33. Have you ever had a seizure? ☐ ☐
34. Do you have headaches with exercise? ☐ ☐
35. Have you ever had numbness, tingling, or weakness in your arms or legs after being hit or falling? ☐ ☐
36. Have you ever been unable to move your arms or legs after being hit or falling? ☐ ☐
37. When exercising in the heat, do you have severe muscle cramps or become ill? ☐ ☐
38. Has a doctor told you that you or someone in your family has sickle cell trait or sickle cell disease? ☐ ☐
39. Have you had any problems with your eyes or vision? ☐ ☐
40. Do you wear glasses or contact lenses? ☐ ☐
41. Do you wear protective eyewear, such as goggles or a face shield? ☐ ☐
42. Are you happy with your weight? ☐ ☐
43. Are you trying to gain or lose weight? ☐ ☐
44. Has anyone recommended you change your weight or eating habits? ☐ ☐
45. Do you limit or carefully control what you eat? ☐ ☐
46. Do you have any concerns that you would like to discuss with a doctor? ☐ ☐

FEMALES ONLY
47. Have you ever had a menstrual period? ☐ ☐
48. How old were you when you had your first menstrual period? _____
49. How many periods have you had in the last 12 months?_____

Explain "Yes" answers here: _____

_____
_____
_____
_____
_____
_____

I hereby state that, to the best of my knowledge, my answers to the above questions are complete and correct.

Signature of athlete _____ Signature of parent/guardian _____ Date _____

Preparticipation Physical Evaluation

Name _____ Date of birth _____

Height _____ Weight_____ % Body fat (optional) _____ Pulse_____ BP___/____ (___/___ , ___/___)

Vision R 20/ _____ L 20/ _____   Corrected: Y N   Pupils: Equal _____ Unequal _____

Follow-Up Questions on More Sensitive Issues	Yes	No
1. Do you feel stressed out or under a lot of pressure?	☐	☐
2. Do you ever feel so sad or hopeless that you stop doing some of your usual activities for more than a few days?	☐	☐
3. Do you feel safe?	☐	☐
4. Have you ever tried cigarette smoking, even 1 or 2 puffs? Do you currently smoke?	☐	☐
5. During the past 30 days, did you use chewing tobacco, snuff, or dip?	☐	☐
6. During the past 30 days, have you had at least 1 drink of alcohol?	☐	☐
7. Have you ever taken steroid pills or shots without a doctor's prescription?	☐	☐
8. Have you ever taken any supplements to help you gain or lose weight or improve your performance?	☐	☐
9. Questions from the Youth Risk Behavior Survey (http://www.cdc.gov/HealthyYouth/yrbs/index.htm) on guns, seatbelts, unprotected sex, domestic violence, drugs, etc.	☐	☐

Notes: _____
_____
_____

	NORMAL	ABNORMAL FINDINGS	INITIALS*
MEDICAL			
Appearance			
Eyes/ears/nose/throat			
Hearing			
Lymph nodes			
Heart			
Murmurs			
Pulses			
Lungs			
Abdomen			
Genitourinary (males only)†			
Skin			
MUSCULOSKELETAL			
Neck			
Back			
Shoulder/arm			
Elbow/forearm			
Wrist/hand/fingers			
Hip/thigh			
Knee			
Leg/ankle			
Foot/toes			

*Multiple-examiner set-up only.
†Having a third party present is recommended for the genitourinary examination.

Notes: _____
_____

Name of physician (print/type) _____ Date _____

Address _____ Phone _____

Signature of physician _____ , MD or DO

Preparticipation Physical Evaluation

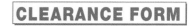

CLEARANCE FORM

Name _____ Sex _____ Age _____ Date of birth _____

❑ **Cleared without restriction**

❑ **Cleared, with recommendations for further evaluation or treatment for:** _____

_____

_____

_____

❑ **Not cleared for**   ❑ **All sports** ❑ **Certain sports:** _____   **Reason:** _____

Recommendations: _____

_____

EMERGENCY INFORMATION

Allergies _____

Other Information _____

IMMUNIZATIONS (eg, tetanus/diphtheria; measles, mumps, rubella; hepatitis A, B; influenza; poliomyelitis; pneumococcal; meningococcal; varicella)

❑ **Up to date (see attached documentation)**   ❑ **Not up to date** Specify _____

Name of physician (print/type) _____ **Date** _____

Address _____ **Phone** _____

Signature of physician _____, **MD or DO**

Preparticipation Physical Evaluation

CLEARANCE FORM

Name _____ Sex _____ Age _____ Date of birth _____

❑ **Cleared without restriction**

❑ **Cleared, with recommendations for further evaluation or treatment for:** _____

_____

_____

_____

❑ **Not cleared for**   ❑ **All sports** ❑ **Certain sports:** _____   **Reason:** _____

Recommendations: _____

_____

EMERGENCY INFORMATION

Allergies _____

Other Information _____

IMMUNIZATIONS (eg, tetanus/diphtheria; measles, mumps, rubella; hepatitis A, B; influenza; poliomyelitis; pneumococcal; meningococcal; varicella)

❑ **Up to date (see attached documentation)**   ❑ **Not up to date** Specify _____

Name of physician (print/type) _____ **Date** _____

Address _____ **Phone** _____

Signature of physician _____, **MD or DO**

Example of a College PPE Consent Form

Consent to Participate in Varsity Athletics

Student Information

Student Name: _____ Birth date: _____ Sex: _____

Address: _____

City, State: _____

Phone: _____

Medical Insurance Company: _____ Policy number: _____

Parent/Guardian and Student Consent

I consent to the participation of the above-named student in varsity athletics, including practice sessions and travel to and from athletic contests. If the medical status of the student changes in any significant manner after passing the physical examination, I will notify the university immediately. I also consent to the use of the data collected in the health questionnaire for research purposes, the results of which will be restricted to sports participation health risk assessment. Release of any information for research purposes, including published results, will not in any way identify the student.

Signature of Parent/Guardian (if student under 18 years) _____ Date: _____

Signature of Student _____ Date: _____

Physician Clearance

I certify that I have on this date examined this student and that, on the basis of the examination requested by the NCAA and the student's medical history as furnished to me, this student is:

CLEARED TO PARTICIPATE WITH:
☐ no restrictions
☐ the following restrictions (explain below):

NOT CLEARED TO PARTICIPATE:
☐ Deferred—may be reconsidered after further evaluation (explain below):
☐ Not fit (give reason below):

Explanations:

Examiner's Signature: _____ Date: _____

Name: _____

Address: _____ Phone: _____

Screen for Teens (12 years old) - Young Adults (20 years old)

In order to help you the best we can, we would like you to answer the questions below. We ask all teenagers these questions because we feel they are things that affect your health and well-being. All of the questions may not fit you. You may leave those that do not apply blank. Please answer the questions alone, away from your parents or friends, so you can be as honest as possible. The questionnaire is not mandatory and if there is any disagreement with some of the questions asked, feel free to discuss these with the physician.

Your answers are a confidential/private part of your medical record. However, for your safety, we are required by law to share information involving physical/sexual abuse and suicide. Every situation is individual and our staff will always talk with you before sharing any of this information.

1. Do you get some exercise at least 3 times a week?	Yes	Sometimes		No
2. Do you wear a seat belt in a car/truck?	Yes	Sometimes		No
3. Do you wear a helmet when you skateboard, bicycle, motorcycle, snowmobile, or use an ATV?	Yes	Sometimes		No
4. How often do you eat a well-balanced diet? A well-balanced diet includes selections from each of these groups: • Fruits and vegetables; • Bread/cereal/rice/pasta; • Milk/yogurt/cheese; and • Meat/poultry/fish/dry beans	Every day	Most days	Some days	Rarely or never
5. Do you use sun block at SPF 15 or greater to protect skin from the sun?	Always	Most of the time	Sometimes	Rarely or never
6. In general, are you happy with the way things are going for you?	Yes	Sometimes		No
7. Do you get along with your family?	Yes	Sometimes		No
8. Do you go to school regularly?	Yes	Sometimes		No
9. Have your grades gotten worse than they used to be?	No			Yes
10. Do you have at least one adult you can really talk to?	Yes	Sometimes		No
11. Do you feel you are about the right weight for your height?	Yes	Sometimes		No
12. Do you ever use laxatives or throw up on purpose after eating?	No	Sometimes		Yes
13. Do you smoke cigarettes or chew tobacco?	No	Sometimes		Yes
14. Do you drink alcohol?	No	Sometimes		Yes
15. Have you tried any drugs (pot, crack, cocaine, heroin, acid, speed, etc)?	No			Yes
16. Do you—or does anyone you live with—have a gun or carry a gun around?	No	Sometimes		Yes
17. Are you—or have you been—in a gang?	No			Yes
18. Are you worried about money, a place to live, or having enough food to eat?	No	Sometimes		Yes
19. Have you ever had sex (with women, men or both)?	No			Yes
20. Have you ever been tested for or diagnosed with a sexually transmitted disease (VD)? (herpes, gonorrhea, Chlamydia, genital warts, PID, syphilis)	No			Yes
21. Are you—or do you ever wonder if you are—gay, lesbian, bisexual, or transgender?	No	Sometimes		Yes
22. How often are you using birth control (such as birth control pills, condoms, diaphragms, or Deproprovera)?	Does not Apply	Always	Sometimes	Never
23. Are you planning a pregnancy or at risk for becoming pregnant?	No	Uncertain		Yes
Please re-read the italicized paragraph at the top before answering the following questions.				
24. Have you ever thought about killing yourself?	No			Yes
25. Do you feel afraid in any of your relationships?	No			Yes
26. Have you ever been physically or sexually abused or mistreated by anyone (kicked, hit, pushed, forced or tricked into having sex, touched on your private parts)?	No			Yes

Adapted with permission from Ramsey Family Physicians Clinic Teen Screen.